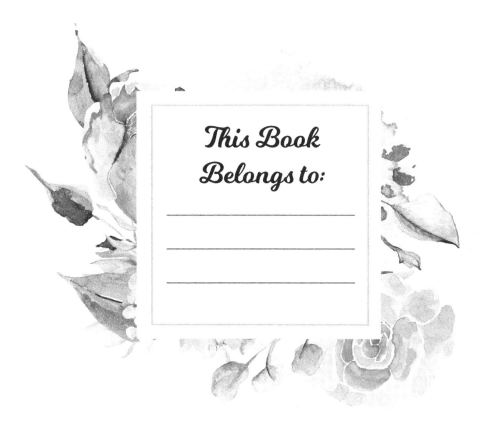

This Book
Belongs to:

_____

_____

_____

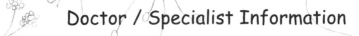

Doctor / Specialist Information

Doctor's Appointments	Date	Doctor's Name	Contact

Dialy Medication / Supplements

Medication / Drugs	Amount

Pain Summary

Entry	Rating	Entry	Rating
1	① ② ③ ④ ⑤ ⑥ ⑦ ⑧ ⑨ ⑩	31	① ② ③ ④ ⑤ ⑥ ⑦ ⑧ ⑨ ⑩
2	① ② ③ ④ ⑤ ⑥ ⑦ ⑧ ⑨ ⑩	32	① ② ③ ④ ⑤ ⑥ ⑦ ⑧ ⑨ ⑩
3	① ② ③ ④ ⑤ ⑥ ⑦ ⑧ ⑨ ⑩	33	① ② ③ ④ ⑤ ⑥ ⑦ ⑧ ⑨ ⑩
4	① ② ③ ④ ⑤ ⑥ ⑦ ⑧ ⑨ ⑩	34	① ② ③ ④ ⑤ ⑥ ⑦ ⑧ ⑨ ⑩
5	① ② ③ ④ ⑤ ⑥ ⑦ ⑧ ⑨ ⑩	35	① ② ③ ④ ⑤ ⑥ ⑦ ⑧ ⑨ ⑩
6	① ② ③ ④ ⑤ ⑥ ⑦ ⑧ ⑨ ⑩	36	① ② ③ ④ ⑤ ⑥ ⑦ ⑧ ⑨ ⑩
7	① ② ③ ④ ⑤ ⑥ ⑦ ⑧ ⑨ ⑩	37	① ② ③ ④ ⑤ ⑥ ⑦ ⑧ ⑨ ⑩
8	① ② ③ ④ ⑤ ⑥ ⑦ ⑧ ⑨ ⑩	38	① ② ③ ④ ⑤ ⑥ ⑦ ⑧ ⑨ ⑩
9	① ② ③ ④ ⑤ ⑥ ⑦ ⑧ ⑨ ⑩	39	① ② ③ ④ ⑤ ⑥ ⑦ ⑧ ⑨ ⑩
10	① ② ③ ④ ⑤ ⑥ ⑦ ⑧ ⑨ ⑩	40	① ② ③ ④ ⑤ ⑥ ⑦ ⑧ ⑨ ⑩
11	① ② ③ ④ ⑤ ⑥ ⑦ ⑧ ⑨ ⑩	41	① ② ③ ④ ⑤ ⑥ ⑦ ⑧ ⑨ ⑩
12	① ② ③ ④ ⑤ ⑥ ⑦ ⑧ ⑨ ⑩	42	① ② ③ ④ ⑤ ⑥ ⑦ ⑧ ⑨ ⑩
13	① ② ③ ④ ⑤ ⑥ ⑦ ⑧ ⑨ ⑩	43	① ② ③ ④ ⑤ ⑥ ⑦ ⑧ ⑨ ⑩
14	① ② ③ ④ ⑤ ⑥ ⑦ ⑧ ⑨ ⑩	44	① ② ③ ④ ⑤ ⑥ ⑦ ⑧ ⑨ ⑩
15	① ② ③ ④ ⑤ ⑥ ⑦ ⑧ ⑨ ⑩	45	① ② ③ ④ ⑤ ⑥ ⑦ ⑧ ⑨ ⑩
16	① ② ③ ④ ⑤ ⑥ ⑦ ⑧ ⑨ ⑩	46	① ② ③ ④ ⑤ ⑥ ⑦ ⑧ ⑨ ⑩
17	① ② ③ ④ ⑤ ⑥ ⑦ ⑧ ⑨ ⑩	47	① ② ③ ④ ⑤ ⑥ ⑦ ⑧ ⑨ ⑩
18	① ② ③ ④ ⑤ ⑥ ⑦ ⑧ ⑨ ⑩	48	① ② ③ ④ ⑤ ⑥ ⑦ ⑧ ⑨ ⑩
19	① ② ③ ④ ⑤ ⑥ ⑦ ⑧ ⑨ ⑩	49	① ② ③ ④ ⑤ ⑥ ⑦ ⑧ ⑨ ⑩
20	① ② ③ ④ ⑤ ⑥ ⑦ ⑧ ⑨ ⑩	50	① ② ③ ④ ⑤ ⑥ ⑦ ⑧ ⑨ ⑩
21	① ② ③ ④ ⑤ ⑥ ⑦ ⑧ ⑨ ⑩	51	① ② ③ ④ ⑤ ⑥ ⑦ ⑧ ⑨ ⑩
22	① ② ③ ④ ⑤ ⑥ ⑦ ⑧ ⑨ ⑩	52	① ② ③ ④ ⑤ ⑥ ⑦ ⑧ ⑨ ⑩
23	① ② ③ ④ ⑤ ⑥ ⑦ ⑧ ⑨ ⑩	53	① ② ③ ④ ⑤ ⑥ ⑦ ⑧ ⑨ ⑩
24	① ② ③ ④ ⑤ ⑥ ⑦ ⑧ ⑨ ⑩	54	① ② ③ ④ ⑤ ⑥ ⑦ ⑧ ⑨ ⑩
25	① ② ③ ④ ⑤ ⑥ ⑦ ⑧ ⑨ ⑩	55	① ② ③ ④ ⑤ ⑥ ⑦ ⑧ ⑨ ⑩
26	① ② ③ ④ ⑤ ⑥ ⑦ ⑧ ⑨ ⑩	56	① ② ③ ④ ⑤ ⑥ ⑦ ⑧ ⑨ ⑩
27	① ② ③ ④ ⑤ ⑥ ⑦ ⑧ ⑨ ⑩	57	① ② ③ ④ ⑤ ⑥ ⑦ ⑧ ⑨ ⑩
28	① ② ③ ④ ⑤ ⑥ ⑦ ⑧ ⑨ ⑩	58	① ② ③ ④ ⑤ ⑥ ⑦ ⑧ ⑨ ⑩
29	① ② ③ ④ ⑤ ⑥ ⑦ ⑧ ⑨ ⑩	59	① ② ③ ④ ⑤ ⑥ ⑦ ⑧ ⑨ ⑩
30	① ② ③ ④ ⑤ ⑥ ⑦ ⑧ ⑨ ⑩	60	① ② ③ ④ ⑤ ⑥ ⑦ ⑧ ⑨ ⑩

Date: _____ Hours of Sleep: _____ Sleep Quality: ⭐☆☆☆☆

Weather: ☀ ☁ ⛅ 🌧 🌦 ❄ Temp: _____

BM Pressure: _____ Allergen Levels: _____

Water: ⊔⊔⊔⊔⊔⊔⊔⊔⊔⊔⊔⊔⊔⊔⊔⊔⊔⊔⊔

Rate Your Pain Level

No Pain (1) (2) (3) (4) (5) (6) (7) (8) (9) (10) Severe pain

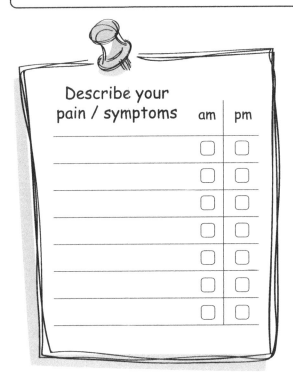

Describe your pain / symptoms

	am	pm
	☐	☐
	☐	☐
	☐	☐
	☐	☐
	☐	☐
	☐	☐
	☐	☐

Where does it hurt?

Front   Back

Mood:	🙂 😖 😣 😍 😴 😓 😟 😠
Energy Level:	(1) (2) (3) (4) (5) (6) (7) (8) (9) (10)
Stress Level:	(1) (2) (3) (4) (5) (6) (7) (8) (9) (10)
Mental Clarity:	(1) (2) (3) (4) (5) (6) (7) (8) (9) (10)

Feeling Sick? ☐ Yes ☐ No

☐ Nausea   ☐ Vomiting   ☐ Congestion   ☐ Fever
☐ Diarrhea   ☐ Sore Throat   ☐ Coughing   ☐ Chills

Medications	Time	Dose

Breakfast:

Lunch:

Dinner:

Snacks:

Exercise

☐ None   ☐ Stretching   ☐ Running/Jogging ☐ Yoga
☐ Walking   ☐ Cardio/Weights   ☐

Notes:

Date: _____ Hours of Sleep: _____ Sleep Quality: ★☆☆☆☆

Weather: ☀ ☁ ⛅ 🌧 🌦 ❄ Temp: _____

BM Pressure: _____ Allergen Levels: _____

Water: ⊔⊔⊔⊔⊔⊔⊔⊔⊔⊔⊔⊔⊔⊔⊔⊔⊔⊔

— Rate Your Pain Level —

No Pain ① ② ③ ④ ⑤ ⑥ ⑦ ⑧ ⑨ ⑩ Severe pain

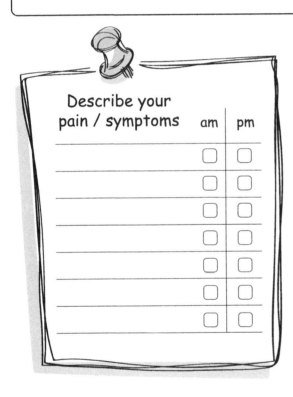

Describe your pain / symptoms

	am	pm
	☐	☐
	☐	☐
	☐	☐
	☐	☐
	☐	☐
	☐	☐
	☐	☐

Where does it hurt?

Front   Back

Mood: 🙂 😣 😭 😍 😴 😓 😧 😠

Energy Level: ① ② ③ ④ ⑤ ⑥ ⑦ ⑧ ⑨ ⑩

Stress Level: ① ② ③ ④ ⑤ ⑥ ⑦ ⑧ ⑨ ⑩

Mental Clarity: ① ② ③ ④ ⑤ ⑥ ⑦ ⑧ ⑨ ⑩

Feeling Sick? ☐ Yes ☐ No

☐ Nausea   ☐ Vomiting   ☐ Congestion   ☐ Fever
☐ Diarrhea   ☐ Sore Throat   ☐ Coughing   ☐ Chills

Medications	Time	Dose

Breakfast:

Lunch:

Dinner:

Snacks:

Exercise

☐ None   ☐ Stretching   ☐ Running/Jogging ☐ Yoga
☐ Walking ☐ Cardio/Weights   ☐

Notes:

Date: _____ Hours of Sleep: _____ Sleep Quality: ★☆☆☆☆

Weather: ☀ ☁ ⛅ 🌧 🌦 ❄ Temp: _____

BM Pressure: _____ Allergen Levels: _____

Water: ▢▢▢▢▢▢▢▢▢▢▢▢▢▢▢▢▢▢

Rate Your Pain Level

No Pain ① ② ③ ④ ⑤ ⑥ ⑦ ⑧ ⑨ ⑩ Severe pain

Describe your pain / symptoms

	am	pm
_____	▢	▢
_____	▢	▢
_____	▢	▢
_____	▢	▢
_____	▢	▢
_____	▢	▢
_____	▢	▢

Where does it hurt?

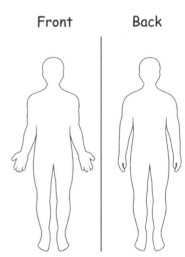

Front   Back

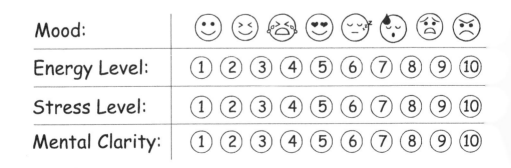

Mood:	🙂 😆 😭 😍 😴 😓 😣 😠
Energy Level:	① ② ③ ④ ⑤ ⑥ ⑦ ⑧ ⑨ ⑩
Stress Level:	① ② ③ ④ ⑤ ⑥ ⑦ ⑧ ⑨ ⑩
Mental Clarity:	① ② ③ ④ ⑤ ⑥ ⑦ ⑧ ⑨ ⑩

Feeling Sick? ☐ Yes ☐ No

☐ Nausea ☐ Vomiting ☐ Congestion ☐ Fever

☐ Diarrhea ☐ Sore Throat ☐ Coughing ☐ Chills

Medications	Time	Dose

Breakfast:

Lunch:

Dinner:

Snacks:

Exercise

☐ None ☐ Stretching ☐ Running/Jogging ☐ Yoga

☐ Walking ☐ Cardio/Weights ☐

Notes:

Date: _____ Hours of Sleep: _____ Sleep Quality: ⭐☆☆☆☆

Weather: ☀ ☁ ⛅ 🌧 🌦 ❄ Temp: _____

BM Pressure: _____ Allergen Levels: _____

Water: ▯▯▯▯▯▯▯▯▯▯▯▯▯▯▯▯▯▯▯

Rate Your Pain Level

No Pain ① ② ③ ④ ⑤ ⑥ ⑦ ⑧ ⑨ ⑩ Severe pain

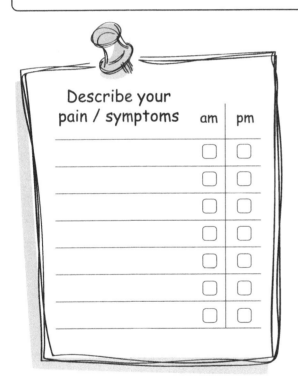

Describe your pain / symptoms

	am	pm
_____	☐	☐
_____	☐	☐
_____	☐	☐
_____	☐	☐
_____	☐	☐
_____	☐	☐
_____	☐	☐

Where does it hurt?

Front   Back

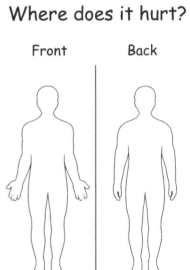

Mood:	🙂 😆 😫 😍 😴 😓 😟 😠
Energy Level:	① ② ③ ④ ⑤ ⑥ ⑦ ⑧ ⑨ ⑩
Stress Level:	① ② ③ ④ ⑤ ⑥ ⑦ ⑧ ⑨ ⑩
Mental Clarity:	① ② ③ ④ ⑤ ⑥ ⑦ ⑧ ⑨ ⑩

Feeling Sick? ☐ Yes ☐ No

☐ Nausea   ☐ Vomiting   ☐ Congestion   ☐ Fever

☐ Diarrhea   ☐ Sore Throat   ☐ Coughing   ☐ Chills

Medications	Time	Dose

Breakfast:

Lunch:

Dinner:

Snacks:

Exercise

☐ None   ☐ Stretching   ☐ Running/Jogging ☐ Yoga

☐ Walking   ☐ Cardio/Weights   ☐

Notes:

Date: _____ Hours of Sleep: _____ Sleep Quality: ★☆☆☆☆

Weather: ☀ ☁ ⛅ 🌧 🌦 ❄ Temp: _____

BM Pressure: _____ Allergen Levels: _____

Water: 🥛🥛🥛🥛🥛🥛🥛🥛🥛🥛🥛🥛🥛🥛🥛🥛🥛

── Rate Your Pain Level ──

No Pain ① ② ③ ④ ⑤ ⑥ ⑦ ⑧ ⑨ ⑩ Severe pain

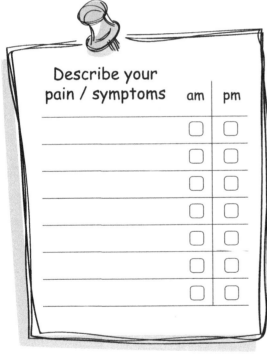

Describe your pain / symptoms

	am	pm
_____	☐	☐
_____	☐	☐
_____	☐	☐
_____	☐	☐
_____	☐	☐
_____	☐	☐
_____	☐	☐

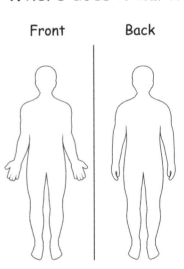

Where does it hurt?

Front   Back

Mood: 🙂 😣 😭 😍 😴 😓 😟 😠

Energy Level: ① ② ③ ④ ⑤ ⑥ ⑦ ⑧ ⑨ ⑩

Stress Level: ① ② ③ ④ ⑤ ⑥ ⑦ ⑧ ⑨ ⑩

Mental Clarity: ① ② ③ ④ ⑤ ⑥ ⑦ ⑧ ⑨ ⑩

Feeling Sick? ☐ Yes ☐ No

☐ Nausea   ☐ Vomiting   ☐ Congestion   ☐ Fever

☐ Diarrhea ☐ Sore Throat ☐ Coughing   ☐ Chills

Medications	Time	Dose

Breakfast:

Lunch:

Dinner:

Snacks:

Exercise

☐ None   ☐ Stretching   ☐ Running/Jogging ☐ Yoga

☐ Walking ☐ Cardio/Weights ☐

Notes:

Date: _____ Hours of Sleep: _____ Sleep Quality: ★☆☆☆☆

Weather: ☀ ☁ ⛅ 🌧 🌦 ❄ Temp: _____

BM Pressure: _____ Allergen Levels: _____

Water: ▢▢▢▢▢▢▢▢▢▢▢▢▢▢▢▢▢▢

Rate Your Pain Level

No Pain ① ② ③ ④ ⑤ ⑥ ⑦ ⑧ ⑨ ⑩ Severe pain

Describe your pain / symptoms

	am	pm
_____	▢	▢
_____	▢	▢
_____	▢	▢
_____	▢	▢
_____	▢	▢
_____	▢	▢
_____	▢	▢

Where does it hurt?

Front   Back

Mood: 🙂 😆 😫 😍 😴 😓 😣 😠

Energy Level: ① ② ③ ④ ⑤ ⑥ ⑦ ⑧ ⑨ ⑩

Stress Level: ① ② ③ ④ ⑤ ⑥ ⑦ ⑧ ⑨ ⑩

Mental Clarity: ① ② ③ ④ ⑤ ⑥ ⑦ ⑧ ⑨ ⑩

Feeling Sick? ☐ Yes ☐ No

☐ Nausea ☐ Vomiting ☐ Congestion ☐ Fever
☐ Diarrhea ☐ Sore Throat ☐ Coughing ☐ Chills

Medications	Time	Dose

Breakfast:

Lunch:

Dinner:

Snacks:

Exercise

☐ None ☐ Stretching ☐ Running/Jogging ☐ Yoga
☐ Walking ☐ Cardio/Weights ☐

Notes:

Date: _____ Hours of Sleep: _____ Sleep Quality: ★☆☆☆☆

Weather: ☀ ☁ ⛅ 🌧 🌦 ❄ Temp: _____

BM Pressure: _____ Allergen Levels: _____

Water: ⊔⊔⊔⊔⊔⊔⊔⊔⊔⊔⊔⊔⊔⊔⊔⊔⊔⊔

Rate Your Pain Level

No Pain ① ② ③ ④ ⑤ ⑥ ⑦ ⑧ ⑨ ⑩ Severe pain

Describe your pain / symptoms

	am	pm
_____	☐	☐
_____	☐	☐
_____	☐	☐
_____	☐	☐
_____	☐	☐
_____	☐	☐
_____	☐	☐

Where does it hurt?

Front   Back

Mood:	🙂 😆 😭 😍 😴 😓 😟 😠
Energy Level:	① ② ③ ④ ⑤ ⑥ ⑦ ⑧ ⑨ ⑩
Stress Level:	① ② ③ ④ ⑤ ⑥ ⑦ ⑧ ⑨ ⑩
Mental Clarity:	① ② ③ ④ ⑤ ⑥ ⑦ ⑧ ⑨ ⑩

Feeling Sick? ☐ Yes ☐ No

☐ Nausea ☐ Vomiting ☐ Congestion ☐ Fever

☐ Diarrhea ☐ Sore Throat ☐ Coughing ☐ Chills

Medications	Time	Dose

Breakfast:

Lunch:

Dinner:

Snacks:

Exercise

☐ None ☐ Stretching ☐ Running/Jogging ☐ Yoga

☐ Walking ☐ Cardio/Weights ☐

Notes:

Date: _____ Hours of Sleep: _____ Sleep Quality: ★☆☆☆☆

Weather: ☀ ☁ ⛅ 🌧 🌦 ❄ Temp: _____

BM Pressure: _____ Allergen Levels: _____

Water: ⊔⊔⊔⊔⊔⊔⊔⊔⊔⊔⊔⊔⊔⊔⊔⊔⊔⊔

——— Rate Your Pain Level ———

No Pain ① ② ③ ④ ⑤ ⑥ ⑦ ⑧ ⑨ ⑩ Severe pain

Describe your pain / symptoms

	am	pm
____	☐	☐
____	☐	☐
____	☐	☐
____	☐	☐
____	☐	☐
____	☐	☐
____	☐	☐

Where does it hurt?

Front   Back

Mood:	😊 😣 😭 😍 😴 😓 😩 😠
Energy Level:	① ② ③ ④ ⑤ ⑥ ⑦ ⑧ ⑨ ⑩
Stress Level:	① ② ③ ④ ⑤ ⑥ ⑦ ⑧ ⑨ ⑩
Mental Clarity:	① ② ③ ④ ⑤ ⑥ ⑦ ⑧ ⑨ ⑩

Feeling Sick? ☐ Yes ☐ No

☐ Nausea ☐ Vomiting ☐ Congestion ☐ Fever

☐ Diarrhea ☐ Sore Throat ☐ Coughing ☐ Chills

Medications	Time	Dose

Breakfast:

Lunch:

Dinner:

Snacks:

Exercise

☐ None ☐ Stretching ☐ Running/Jogging ☐ Yoga

☐ Walking ☐ Cardio/Weights ☐

Notes:

Date: _____ Hours of Sleep: _____ Sleep Quality: ★☆☆☆☆

Weather: ☀ ☁ ⛅ 🌧 🌦 ❄ Temp: _____

BM Pressure: _____ Allergen Levels: _____

Water: 🥤🥤🥤🥤🥤🥤🥤🥤🥤🥤🥤🥤🥤🥤🥤🥤🥤🥤

Rate Your Pain Level

No Pain (1) (2) (3) (4) (5) (6) (7) (8) (9) (10) Severe pain

Describe your pain / symptoms

	am	pm
_____	☐	☐
_____	☐	☐
_____	☐	☐
_____	☐	☐
_____	☐	☐
_____	☐	☐
_____	☐	☐

Where does it hurt?

Front   Back

Mood:	🙂 😆 😭 😍 😴 🥵 😣 😠
Energy Level:	(1) (2) (3) (4) (5) (6) (7) (8) (9) (10)
Stress Level:	(1) (2) (3) (4) (5) (6) (7) (8) (9) (10)
Mental Clarity:	(1) (2) (3) (4) (5) (6) (7) (8) (9) (10)

Feeling Sick? ☐ Yes ☐ No

☐ Nausea   ☐ Vomiting   ☐ Congestion   ☐ Fever
☐ Diarrhea   ☐ Sore Throat   ☐ Coughing   ☐ Chills

Medications	Time	Dose

Breakfast:

Lunch:

Dinner:

Snacks:

Exercise

☐ None   ☐ Stretching   ☐ Running/Jogging   ☐ Yoga
☐ Walking   ☐ Cardio/Weights   ☐

Notes:

Date: _____ Hours of Sleep: _____ Sleep Quality: ★☆☆☆☆

Weather: ☀ ☁ ⛅ 🌧 🌦 ❄ Temp: _____

BM Pressure: _____ Allergen Levels: _____

Water: 🥛🥛🥛🥛🥛🥛🥛🥛🥛🥛🥛🥛🥛🥛🥛🥛

Rate Your Pain Level

No Pain ① ② ③ ④ ⑤ ⑥ ⑦ ⑧ ⑨ ⑩ Severe pain

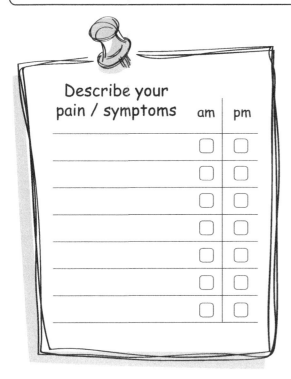

Describe your pain / symptoms · am · pm

Where does it hurt?
Front · Back

Mood:	🙂 😣 😭 😍 😴 😓 😧 😠
Energy Level:	① ② ③ ④ ⑤ ⑥ ⑦ ⑧ ⑨ ⑩
Stress Level:	① ② ③ ④ ⑤ ⑥ ⑦ ⑧ ⑨ ⑩
Mental Clarity:	① ② ③ ④ ⑤ ⑥ ⑦ ⑧ ⑨ ⑩

Feeling Sick? ☐ Yes ☐ No

☐ Nausea ☐ Vomiting ☐ Congestion ☐ Fever

☐ Diarrhea ☐ Sore Throat ☐ Coughing ☐ Chills

Medications	Time	Dose

Breakfast:

Lunch:

Dinner:

Snacks:

Exercise

☐ None ☐ Stretching ☐ Running/Jogging ☐ Yoga

☐ Walking ☐ Cardio/Weights ☐

Notes:

Date: _____ Hours of Sleep: _____ Sleep Quality: ★☆☆☆☆

Weather: ☀ ☁ ⛅ 🌧 🌦 ❄ Temp: _____

BM Pressure: _____ Allergen Levels: _____

Water:

— Rate Your Pain Level —

No Pain ① ② ③ ④ ⑤ ⑥ ⑦ ⑧ ⑨ ⑩ Severe pain

Describe your pain / symptoms | am | pm

Where does it hurt?

Front   Back

Mood: 😊 😆 😭 😍 😴 😰 😖 😠

Energy Level: ① ② ③ ④ ⑤ ⑥ ⑦ ⑧ ⑨ ⑩

Stress Level: ① ② ③ ④ ⑤ ⑥ ⑦ ⑧ ⑨ ⑩

Mental Clarity: ① ② ③ ④ ⑤ ⑥ ⑦ ⑧ ⑨ ⑩

Feeling Sick? ☐ Yes ☐ No

☐ Nausea   ☐ Vomiting   ☐ Congestion   ☐ Fever

☐ Diarrhea   ☐ Sore Throat   ☐ Coughing   ☐ Chills

Medications	Time	Dose

Breakfast:

Lunch:

Dinner:

Snacks:

Exercise

☐ None   ☐ Stretching   ☐ Running/Jogging ☐ Yoga

☐ Walking ☐ Cardio/Weights   ☐

Notes:

Date: _____ Hours of Sleep: _____ Sleep Quality: ★☆☆☆☆

Weather: ☀ ☁ ⛅ 🌧 🌦 ❄ Temp: _____

BM Pressure: _____ Allergen Levels: _____

Water: 🥛🥛🥛🥛🥛🥛🥛🥛🥛🥛🥛🥛🥛🥛🥛🥛🥛

Rate Your Pain Level

No Pain (1) (2) (3) (4) (5) (6) (7) (8) (9) (10) Severe pain

Describe your pain / symptoms

	am	pm
	☐	☐
	☐	☐
	☐	☐
	☐	☐
	☐	☐
	☐	☐
	☐	☐

Where does it hurt?

Front   Back

Mood:	🙂 😆 😭 😍 😴 🥵 😟 😠
Energy Level:	(1) (2) (3) (4) (5) (6) (7) (8) (9) (10)
Stress Level:	(1) (2) (3) (4) (5) (6) (7) (8) (9) (10)
Mental Clarity:	(1) (2) (3) (4) (5) (6) (7) (8) (9) (10)

Feeling Sick? ☐ Yes ☐ No

☐ Nausea ☐ Vomiting ☐ Congestion ☐ Fever
☐ Diarrhea ☐ Sore Throat ☐ Coughing ☐ Chills

Medications	Time	Dose

Breakfast:

Lunch:

Dinner:

Snacks:

Exercise

☐ None ☐ Stretching ☐ Running/Jogging ☐ Yoga
☐ Walking ☐ Cardio/Weights ☐

Notes:

（13）

Date: _____ Hours of Sleep: _____ Sleep Quality: ★☆☆☆☆

Weather: ☀ ☁ ⛅ 🌧 🌦 ❄ Temp: _____

BM Pressure: _____ Allergen Levels: _____

Water: ▢▢▢▢▢▢▢▢▢▢▢▢▢▢▢▢▢▢▢

— Rate Your Pain Level —

No Pain ① ② ③ ④ ⑤ ⑥ ⑦ ⑧ ⑨ ⑩ Severe pain

Describe your pain / symptoms

	am	pm
_____	☐	☐
_____	☐	☐
_____	☐	☐
_____	☐	☐
_____	☐	☐
_____	☐	☐
_____	☐	☐

Where does it hurt?

Front　　　Back

Mood:	🙂 😖 😭 😍 😴 😓 😣 😠
Energy Level:	① ② ③ ④ ⑤ ⑥ ⑦ ⑧ ⑨ ⑩
Stress Level:	① ② ③ ④ ⑤ ⑥ ⑦ ⑧ ⑨ ⑩
Mental Clarity:	① ② ③ ④ ⑤ ⑥ ⑦ ⑧ ⑨ ⑩

Feeling Sick? ☐ Yes ☐ No

☐ Nausea   ☐ Vomiting   ☐ Congestion   ☐ Fever

☐ Diarrhea ☐ Sore Throat ☐ Coughing   ☐ Chills

Medications	Time	Dose

Breakfast:

Lunch:

Dinner:

Snacks:

Exercise

☐ None   ☐ Stretching   ☐ Running/Jogging ☐ Yoga

☐ Walking ☐ Cardio/Weights ☐

Notes:

Date: _____ Hours of Sleep: _____ Sleep Quality: ★☆☆☆☆

Weather: ☀ ☁ ⛅ 🌧 🌦 ❄ Temp: _____

BM Pressure: _____ Allergen Levels: _____

Water: ⊔⊔⊔⊔⊔⊔⊔⊔⊔⊔⊔⊔⊔⊔⊔⊔⊔⊔

Rate Your Pain Level

No Pain ① ② ③ ④ ⑤ ⑥ ⑦ ⑧ ⑨ ⑩ Severe pain

Describe your pain / symptoms

	am	pm
	☐	☐
	☐	☐
	☐	☐
	☐	☐
	☐	☐
	☐	☐
	☐	☐

Where does it hurt?

Front   Back

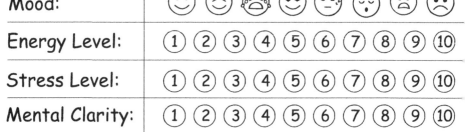

Mood:	🙂 😆 😣 😍 😴 😓 😟 😠
Energy Level:	① ② ③ ④ ⑤ ⑥ ⑦ ⑧ ⑨ ⑩
Stress Level:	① ② ③ ④ ⑤ ⑥ ⑦ ⑧ ⑨ ⑩
Mental Clarity:	① ② ③ ④ ⑤ ⑥ ⑦ ⑧ ⑨ ⑩

Feeling Sick? ☐ Yes ☐ No

☐ Nausea ☐ Vomiting ☐ Congestion ☐ Fever

☐ Diarrhea ☐ Sore Throat ☐ Coughing ☐ Chills

Medications	Time	Dose

Breakfast:

Lunch:

Dinner:

Snacks:

Exercise

☐ None ☐ Stretching ☐ Running/Jogging ☐ Yoga

☐ Walking ☐ Cardio/Weights ☐

Notes:

Date: _____ Hours of Sleep: _____ Sleep Quality: ★☆☆☆☆

Weather: ☀ ☁ ⛅ 🌧 🌦 ❄ Temp: _____

BM Pressure: _____ Allergen Levels: _____

Water: ⬜⬜⬜⬜⬜⬜⬜⬜⬜⬜⬜⬜⬜⬜⬜⬜

Rate Your Pain Level

No Pain ① ② ③ ④ ⑤ ⑥ ⑦ ⑧ ⑨ ⑩ Severe pain

Describe your pain / symptoms

	am	pm
_____	☐	☐
_____	☐	☐
_____	☐	☐
_____	☐	☐
_____	☐	☐
_____	☐	☐
_____	☐	☐

Where does it hurt?

Front   Back

Mood:	😊 😆 😭 😍 😴 😓 😣 😠
Energy Level:	① ② ③ ④ ⑤ ⑥ ⑦ ⑧ ⑨ ⑩
Stress Level:	① ② ③ ④ ⑤ ⑥ ⑦ ⑧ ⑨ ⑩
Mental Clarity:	① ② ③ ④ ⑤ ⑥ ⑦ ⑧ ⑨ ⑩

Feeling Sick? ☐ Yes ☐ No

☐ Nausea   ☐ Vomiting   ☐ Congestion   ☐ Fever

☐ Diarrhea   ☐ Sore Throat   ☐ Coughing   ☐ Chills

Medications	Time	Dose

Breakfast:

Lunch:

Dinner:

Snacks:

Exercise

☐ None   ☐ Stretching   ☐ Running/Jogging ☐ Yoga

☐ Walking   ☐ Cardio/Weights ☐

Notes:

Date: _____ Hours of Sleep: _____ Sleep Quality: ★☆☆☆☆

Weather: ☀ ☁ ⛅ 🌧 🌦 ❄ Temp: _____

BM Pressure: _____ Allergen Levels: _____

Water: ⊔⊔⊔⊔⊔⊔⊔⊔⊔⊔⊔⊔⊔⊔⊔⊔⊔⊔⊔⊔

Rate Your Pain Level

No Pain ① ② ③ ④ ⑤ ⑥ ⑦ ⑧ ⑨ ⑩ Severe pain

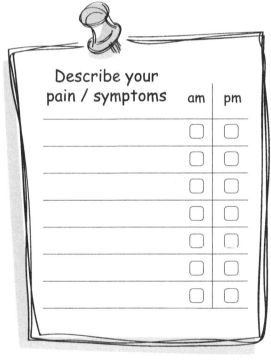

Describe your pain / symptoms	am	pm
_____	☐	☐
_____	☐	☐
_____	☐	☐
_____	☐	☐
_____	☐	☐
_____	☐	☐
_____	☐	☐

Where does it hurt?

Front   Back

Mood: 🙂 😣 😭 😍 😌 😓 ☹ 😠

Energy Level: ① ② ③ ④ ⑤ ⑥ ⑦ ⑧ ⑨ ⑩

Stress Level: ① ② ③ ④ ⑤ ⑥ ⑦ ⑧ ⑨ ⑩

Mental Clarity: ① ② ③ ④ ⑤ ⑥ ⑦ ⑧ ⑨ ⑩

Feeling Sick? ☐ Yes ☐ No

☐ Nausea   ☐ Vomiting   ☐ Congestion   ☐ Fever

☐ Diarrhea   ☐ Sore Throat   ☐ Coughing   ☐ Chills

Medications	Time	Dose

Breakfast:

Lunch:

Dinner:

Snacks:

Exercise

☐ None   ☐ Stretching   ☐ Running/Jogging ☐ Yoga

☐ Walking   ☐ Cardio/Weights   ☐

Notes:

Date: _____ Hours of Sleep: _____ Sleep Quality: ★☆☆☆☆

Weather: ☼ ☁ ⛅ 🌧 🌦 ❄ Temp: _____

BM Pressure: _____ Allergen Levels: _____

Water: ⊔⊔⊔⊔⊔⊔⊔⊔⊔⊔⊔⊔⊔⊔⊔⊔⊔⊔

Rate Your Pain Level

No Pain ① ② ③ ④ ⑤ ⑥ ⑦ ⑧ ⑨ ⑩ Severe pain

Describe your pain / symptoms

	am	pm
_____	☐	☐
_____	☐	☐
_____	☐	☐
_____	☐	☐
_____	☐	☐
_____	☐	☐
_____	☐	☐

Where does it hurt?

Front   Back

Mood:	☺ 😆 😣 😍 😌 😓 😟 😠
Energy Level:	① ② ③ ④ ⑤ ⑥ ⑦ ⑧ ⑨ ⑩
Stress Level:	① ② ③ ④ ⑤ ⑥ ⑦ ⑧ ⑨ ⑩
Mental Clarity:	① ② ③ ④ ⑤ ⑥ ⑦ ⑧ ⑨ ⑩

Feeling Sick? ☐ Yes ☐ No

☐ Nausea   ☐ Vomiting   ☐ Congestion   ☐ Fever

☐ Diarrhea   ☐ Sore Throat   ☐ Coughing   ☐ Chills

Medications	Time	Dose

Breakfast:

Lunch:

Dinner:

Snacks:

Exercise

☐ None   ☐ Stretching   ☐ Running/Jogging ☐ Yoga

☐ Walking ☐ Cardio/Weights ☐

Notes:

Date: _____ Hours of Sleep: _____ Sleep Quality: ★☆☆☆☆

Weather: ☀ ☁ ⛅ 🌧 🌦 ❄ Temp: _____

BM Pressure: _____ Allergen Levels: _____

Water: ⛶⛶⛶⛶⛶⛶⛶⛶⛶⛶⛶⛶⛶⛶⛶⛶

Rate Your Pain Level

No Pain ① ② ③ ④ ⑤ ⑥ ⑦ ⑧ ⑨ ⑩ Severe pain

Describe your pain / symptoms	am	pm
_____	☐	☐
_____	☐	☐
_____	☐	☐
_____	☐	☐
_____	☐	☐
_____	☐	☐
_____	☐	☐

Where does it hurt?

Front   Back

Mood:	😊 😣 😭 😍 😴 😓 😩 😠
Energy Level:	① ② ③ ④ ⑤ ⑥ ⑦ ⑧ ⑨ ⑩
Stress Level:	① ② ③ ④ ⑤ ⑥ ⑦ ⑧ ⑨ ⑩
Mental Clarity:	① ② ③ ④ ⑤ ⑥ ⑦ ⑧ ⑨ ⑩

Feeling Sick? ☐ Yes ☐ No

☐ Nausea   ☐ Vomiting   ☐ Congestion   ☐ Fever
☐ Diarrhea ☐ Sore Throat   ☐ Coughing   ☐ Chills

Medications	Time	Dose

Breakfast:

Lunch:

Dinner:

Snacks:

Exercise

☐ None   ☐ Stretching   ☐ Running/Jogging ☐ Yoga
☐ Walking   ☐ Cardio/Weights   ☐

Notes:

Date: _____   Hours of Sleep: _____   Sleep Quality: ★☆☆☆☆

Weather: ☀ ☁ ⛅ 🌧 🌦 ❄   Temp: _____

BM Pressure: _____   Allergen Levels: _____

Water: ⊔⊔⊔⊔⊔⊔⊔⊔⊔⊔⊔⊔⊔⊔⊔⊔⊔⊔

Rate Your Pain Level

No Pain ① ② ③ ④ ⑤ ⑥ ⑦ ⑧ ⑨ ⑩ Severe pain

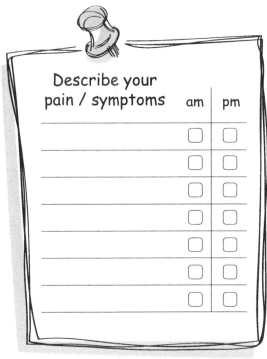

Describe your pain / symptoms   am pm

Where does it hurt?

Front   Back

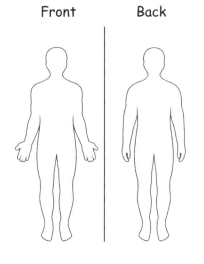

Mood: 🙂 😝 😣 😍 😴 😓 😩 😠

Energy Level: ① ② ③ ④ ⑤ ⑥ ⑦ ⑧ ⑨ ⑩

Stress Level: ① ② ③ ④ ⑤ ⑥ ⑦ ⑧ ⑨ ⑩

Mental Clarity: ① ② ③ ④ ⑤ ⑥ ⑦ ⑧ ⑨ ⑩

Feeling Sick? ☐ Yes ☐ No

☐ Nausea   ☐ Vomiting   ☐ Congestion   ☐ Fever
☐ Diarrhea   ☐ Sore Throat   ☐ Coughing   ☐ Chills

Medications	Time	Dose

Breakfast:

Lunch:

Dinner:

Snacks:

Exercise

☐ None   ☐ Stretching   ☐ Running/Jogging ☐ Yoga
☐ Walking   ☐ Cardio/Weights   ☐

Notes:

Date: _____ Hours of Sleep: _____ Sleep Quality: ★☆☆☆☆

Weather: ☀ ☁ ⛅ 🌧 🌦 ❄ Temp: _____

BM Pressure: _____ Allergen Levels: _____

Water: ▯▯▯▯▯▯▯▯▯▯▯▯▯▯▯▯▯

Rate Your Pain Level

No Pain ① ② ③ ④ ⑤ ⑥ ⑦ ⑧ ⑨ ⑩ Severe pain

Describe your pain / symptoms

	am	pm
_____	☐	☐
_____	☐	☐
_____	☐	☐
_____	☐	☐
_____	☐	☐
_____	☐	☐
_____	☐	☐

Where does it hurt?

Front   Back

Mood: 😊 😆 😫 😍 😴 😓 😧 😠

Energy Level: ① ② ③ ④ ⑤ ⑥ ⑦ ⑧ ⑨ ⑩

Stress Level: ① ② ③ ④ ⑤ ⑥ ⑦ ⑧ ⑨ ⑩

Mental Clarity: ① ② ③ ④ ⑤ ⑥ ⑦ ⑧ ⑨ ⑩

Feeling Sick? ☐ Yes ☐ No

☐ Nausea ☐ Vomiting ☐ Congestion ☐ Fever

☐ Diarrhea ☐ Sore Throat ☐ Coughing ☐ Chills

Medications	Time	Dose

Breakfast:

Lunch:

Dinner:

Snacks:

Exercise

☐ None ☐ Stretching ☐ Running/Jogging ☐ Yoga

☐ Walking ☐ Cardio/Weights ☐

Notes:

Date: _____ Hours of Sleep: _____ Sleep Quality: ★☆☆☆☆

Weather: ☀ ☁ ⛅ 🌧 🌦 ❄ Temp: _____

BM Pressure: _____ Allergen Levels: _____

Water: ⊔⊔⊔⊔⊔⊔⊔⊔⊔⊔⊔⊔⊔⊔⊔⊔⊔

Rate Your Pain Level

No Pain (1) (2) (3) (4) (5) (6) (7) (8) (9) (10) Severe pain

Describe your pain / symptoms

	am	pm
_____	☐	☐
_____	☐	☐
_____	☐	☐
_____	☐	☐
_____	☐	☐
_____	☐	☐
_____	☐	☐

Where does it hurt?

Front   Back

Mood: 🙂 😆 😭 😍 😴 😓 😣 😠

Energy Level: (1) (2) (3) (4) (5) (6) (7) (8) (9) (10)

Stress Level: (1) (2) (3) (4) (5) (6) (7) (8) (9) (10)

Mental Clarity: (1) (2) (3) (4) (5) (6) (7) (8) (9) (10)

Feeling Sick? ☐ Yes ☐ No

☐ Nausea   ☐ Vomiting   ☐ Congestion   ☐ Fever
☐ Diarrhea ☐ Sore Throat ☐ Coughing   ☐ Chills

Medications	Time	Dose

Breakfast:

Lunch:

Dinner:

Snacks:

Exercise

☐ None   ☐ Stretching   ☐ Running/Jogging ☐ Yoga
☐ Walking ☐ Cardio/Weights ☐

Notes:

Date: _____ Hours of Sleep: _____ Sleep Quality: ★☆☆☆☆

Weather: ☀ ☁ ⛅ 🌧 🌦 ❄ Temp: _____

BM Pressure: _____ Allergen Levels: _____

Water: 🥛🥛🥛🥛🥛🥛🥛🥛🥛🥛🥛🥛🥛🥛🥛🥛🥛

——— Rate Your Pain Level ———

No Pain ① ② ③ ④ ⑤ ⑥ ⑦ ⑧ ⑨ ⑩ Severe pain

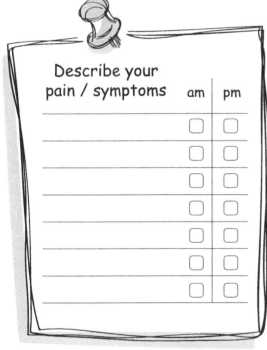

Describe your pain / symptoms

	am	pm
_____	☐	☐
_____	☐	☐
_____	☐	☐
_____	☐	☐
_____	☐	☐
_____	☐	☐
_____	☐	☐

Where does it hurt?

Front   Back

Mood: 😊 😆 😫 😍 😔 😰 😟 😠

Energy Level: ① ② ③ ④ ⑤ ⑥ ⑦ ⑧ ⑨ ⑩

Stress Level: ① ② ③ ④ ⑤ ⑥ ⑦ ⑧ ⑨ ⑩

Mental Clarity: ① ② ③ ④ ⑤ ⑥ ⑦ ⑧ ⑨ ⑩

Feeling Sick? ☐ Yes ☐ No

☐ Nausea   ☐ Vomiting   ☐ Congestion   ☐ Fever

☐ Diarrhea   ☐ Sore Throat   ☐ Coughing   ☐ Chills

Medications	Time	Dose

Breakfast:

Lunch:

Dinner:

Snacks:

Exercise

☐ None   ☐ Stretching   ☐ Running/Jogging ☐ Yoga

☐ Walking   ☐ Cardio/Weights   ☐

Notes:

Date: _____ Hours of Sleep: _____ Sleep Quality: ★☆☆☆☆

Weather: ☀ ☁ ⛅ 🌧 🌦 ❄ Temp: _____

BM Pressure: _____ Allergen Levels: _____

Water: ⊔⊔⊔⊔⊔⊔⊔⊔⊔⊔⊔⊔⊔⊔⊔⊔⊔⊔

Rate Your Pain Level

No Pain ① ② ③ ④ ⑤ ⑥ ⑦ ⑧ ⑨ ⑩ Severe pain

Describe your pain / symptoms

	am	pm
	☐	☐
	☐	☐
	☐	☐
	☐	☐
	☐	☐
	☐	☐
	☐	☐

Where does it hurt?

Front   Back

Mood:	😊 😝 😫 😍 😴 😓 😣 😠
Energy Level:	① ② ③ ④ ⑤ ⑥ ⑦ ⑧ ⑨ ⑩
Stress Level:	① ② ③ ④ ⑤ ⑥ ⑦ ⑧ ⑨ ⑩
Mental Clarity:	① ② ③ ④ ⑤ ⑥ ⑦ ⑧ ⑨ ⑩

Feeling Sick? ☐ Yes ☐ No

☐ Nausea   ☐ Vomiting   ☐ Congestion   ☐ Fever

☐ Diarrhea   ☐ Sore Throat   ☐ Coughing   ☐ Chills

Medications	Time	Dose

Breakfast:

Lunch:

Dinner:

Snacks:

Exercise

☐ None   ☐ Stretching   ☐ Running/Jogging ☐ Yoga

☐ Walking   ☐ Cardio/Weights   ☐

Notes:

Date: _____ Hours of Sleep: _____ Sleep Quality: ★☆☆☆☆

Weather: ☀ ☁ ⛅ 🌧 🌦 ❄ Temp: _____

BM Pressure: _____ Allergen Levels: _____

Water: ⬜⬜⬜⬜⬜⬜⬜⬜⬜⬜⬜⬜⬜⬜⬜⬜⬜

Rate Your Pain Level

No Pain ① ② ③ ④ ⑤ ⑥ ⑦ ⑧ ⑨ ⑩ Severe pain

Describe your pain / symptoms

	am	pm
_____	☐	☐
_____	☐	☐
_____	☐	☐
_____	☐	☐
_____	☐	☐
_____	☐	☐
_____	☐	☐

Where does it hurt?

Front   Back

Mood:	😊 😆 😭 😍 😴 😓 😣 😠
Energy Level:	① ② ③ ④ ⑤ ⑥ ⑦ ⑧ ⑨ ⑩
Stress Level:	① ② ③ ④ ⑤ ⑥ ⑦ ⑧ ⑨ ⑩
Mental Clarity:	① ② ③ ④ ⑤ ⑥ ⑦ ⑧ ⑨ ⑩

Feeling Sick? ☐ Yes ☐ No

☐ Nausea   ☐ Vomiting   ☐ Congestion   ☐ Fever

☐ Diarrhea   ☐ Sore Throat   ☐ Coughing   ☐ Chills

Medications	Time	Dose

Breakfast:

Lunch:

Dinner:

Snacks:

Exercise

☐ None   ☐ Stretching   ☐ Running/Jogging ☐ Yoga

☐ Walking   ☐ Cardio/Weights   ☐

Notes:

Date: _____ Hours of Sleep: _____ Sleep Quality: ★☆☆☆☆

Weather: ☼ ☁ ⛅ 🌧 🌦 ❄ Temp: _____

BM Pressure: _____ Allergen Levels: _____

Water: 🥛🥛🥛🥛🥛🥛🥛🥛🥛🥛🥛🥛🥛🥛🥛🥛🥛

Rate Your Pain Level

No Pain ① ② ③ ④ ⑤ ⑥ ⑦ ⑧ ⑨ ⑩ Severe pain

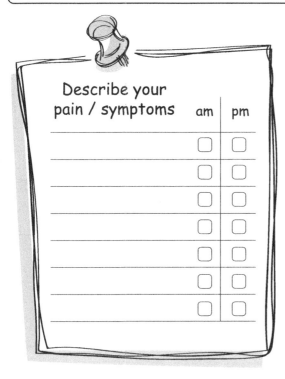

Describe your pain / symptoms   am   pm

Where does it hurt?

Front   Back

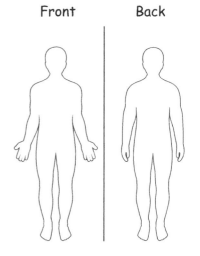

Mood:	🙂 😆 😣 😍 😴 😓 😧 😠
Energy Level:	① ② ③ ④ ⑤ ⑥ ⑦ ⑧ ⑨ ⑩
Stress Level:	① ② ③ ④ ⑤ ⑥ ⑦ ⑧ ⑨ ⑩
Mental Clarity:	① ② ③ ④ ⑤ ⑥ ⑦ ⑧ ⑨ ⑩

Feeling Sick? ☐ Yes ☐ No

☐ Nausea ☐ Vomiting ☐ Congestion ☐ Fever

☐ Diarrhea ☐ Sore Throat ☐ Coughing ☐ Chills

Medications	Time	Dose

Breakfast:

Lunch:

Dinner:

Snacks:

Exercise

☐ None ☐ Stretching ☐ Running/Jogging ☐ Yoga

☐ Walking ☐ Cardio/Weights ☐

Notes:

Date: _____ Hours of Sleep: _____ Sleep Quality: ★☆☆☆☆

Weather: ☀ ☁ ⛅ 🌧 🌦 ❄ Temp: _____

BM Pressure: _____ Allergen Levels: _____

Water: ⬜⬜⬜⬜⬜⬜⬜⬜⬜⬜⬜⬜⬜⬜⬜⬜

Rate Your Pain Level

No Pain ① ② ③ ④ ⑤ ⑥ ⑦ ⑧ ⑨ ⑩ Severe pain

Describe your pain / symptoms

	am	pm
	☐	☐
	☐	☐
	☐	☐
	☐	☐
	☐	☐
	☐	☐
	☐	☐

Where does it hurt?

Front   Back

Mood: 🙂 😝 😫 😍 😴 😰 😣 😠

Energy Level: ① ② ③ ④ ⑤ ⑥ ⑦ ⑧ ⑨ ⑩

Stress Level: ① ② ③ ④ ⑤ ⑥ ⑦ ⑧ ⑨ ⑩

Mental Clarity: ① ② ③ ④ ⑤ ⑥ ⑦ ⑧ ⑨ ⑩

Feeling Sick? ☐ Yes ☐ No

☐ Nausea   ☐ Vomiting   ☐ Congestion   ☐ Fever

☐ Diarrhea   ☐ Sore Throat   ☐ Coughing   ☐ Chills

Medications	Time	Dose

Breakfast:

Lunch:

Dinner:

Snacks:

Exercise

☐ None   ☐ Stretching   ☐ Running/Jogging ☐ Yoga

☐ Walking   ☐ Cardio/Weights   ☐

Notes:

Date: _____ Hours of Sleep: _____ Sleep Quality: ★☆☆☆☆

Weather: ☀ ☁ ⛅ 🌧 🌦 ❄ Temp: _____

BM Pressure: _____ Allergen Levels: _____

Water: ⊔⊔⊔⊔⊔⊔⊔⊔⊔⊔⊔⊔⊔⊔⊔⊔⊔⊔

———— Rate Your Pain Level ————

No Pain ① ② ③ ④ ⑤ ⑥ ⑦ ⑧ ⑨ ⑩ Severe pain

Describe your pain / symptoms

	am	pm
_____	☐	☐
_____	☐	☐
_____	☐	☐
_____	☐	☐
_____	☐	☐
_____	☐	☐
_____	☐	☐

Where does it hurt?

Front   Back

Mood: 😊 😆 😫 😍 😴 😥 😟 😠

Energy Level: ① ② ③ ④ ⑤ ⑥ ⑦ ⑧ ⑨ ⑩

Stress Level: ① ② ③ ④ ⑤ ⑥ ⑦ ⑧ ⑨ ⑩

Mental Clarity: ① ② ③ ④ ⑤ ⑥ ⑦ ⑧ ⑨ ⑩

Feeling Sick? ☐ Yes ☐ No

☐ Nausea ☐ Vomiting ☐ Congestion ☐ Fever

☐ Diarrhea ☐ Sore Throat ☐ Coughing ☐ Chills

Medications	Time	Dose

Breakfast:

Lunch:

Dinner:

Snacks:

Exercise

☐ None ☐ Stretching ☐ Running/Jogging ☐ Yoga

☐ Walking ☐ Cardio/Weights ☐

Notes:

Date: _____ Hours of Sleep: _____ Sleep Quality: ★☆☆☆☆

Weather: ☀ ☁ ⛅ 🌧 🌦 ❄ Temp: _____

BM Pressure: _____ Allergen Levels: _____

Water: ⊔⊔⊔⊔⊔⊔⊔⊔⊔⊔⊔⊔⊔⊔⊔⊔⊔⊔⊔⊔

─── Rate Your Pain Level ───

No Pain ① ② ③ ④ ⑤ ⑥ ⑦ ⑧ ⑨ ⑩ Severe pain

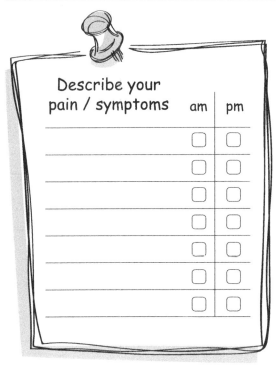

Describe your pain / symptoms

	am	pm
_____	☐	☐
_____	☐	☐
_____	☐	☐
_____	☐	☐
_____	☐	☐
_____	☐	☐
_____	☐	☐

Where does it hurt?

Front   Back

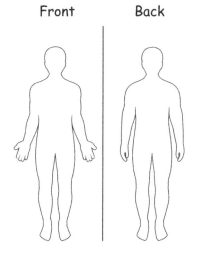

Mood: 🙂 😆 😫 😍 😌 😓 😣 😠

Energy Level: ① ② ③ ④ ⑤ ⑥ ⑦ ⑧ ⑨ ⑩

Stress Level: ① ② ③ ④ ⑤ ⑥ ⑦ ⑧ ⑨ ⑩

Mental Clarity: ① ② ③ ④ ⑤ ⑥ ⑦ ⑧ ⑨ ⑩

Feeling Sick? ☐ Yes ☐ No

☐ Nausea   ☐ Vomiting   ☐ Congestion   ☐ Fever

☐ Diarrhea   ☐ Sore Throat   ☐ Coughing   ☐ Chills

Medications	Time	Dose

Breakfast:

Lunch:

Dinner:

Snacks:

Exercise

☐ None   ☐ Stretching   ☐ Running/Jogging ☐ Yoga

☐ Walking   ☐ Cardio/Weights   ☐

Notes:

Date: _____ Hours of Sleep: _____ Sleep Quality: ★☆☆☆☆

Weather: ☼ ☁ ⛅ 🌧 🌦 ❄ Temp: _____

BM Pressure: _____ Allergen Levels: _____

Water: ▯▯▯▯▯▯▯▯▯▯▯▯▯▯▯▯

Rate Your Pain Level

No Pain ① ② ③ ④ ⑤ ⑥ ⑦ ⑧ ⑨ ⑩ Severe pain

Describe your pain / symptoms

	am	pm
_____	☐	☐
_____	☐	☐
_____	☐	☐
_____	☐	☐
_____	☐	☐
_____	☐	☐
_____	☐	☐

Where does it hurt?

Front   Back

Mood: 😊 😣 😫 😍 😴 😓 😧 😠

Energy Level: ① ② ③ ④ ⑤ ⑥ ⑦ ⑧ ⑨ ⑩

Stress Level: ① ② ③ ④ ⑤ ⑥ ⑦ ⑧ ⑨ ⑩

Mental Clarity: ① ② ③ ④ ⑤ ⑥ ⑦ ⑧ ⑨ ⑩

Feeling Sick? ☐ Yes ☐ No

☐ Nausea   ☐ Vomiting   ☐ Congestion   ☐ Fever

☐ Diarrhea   ☐ Sore Throat   ☐ Coughing   ☐ Chills

Medications	Time	Dose

Breakfast:

Lunch:

Dinner:

Snacks:

Exercise

☐ None   ☐ Stretching   ☐ Running/Jogging ☐ Yoga

☐ Walking   ☐ Cardio/Weights   ☐

Notes:

Date: _____ Hours of Sleep: _____ Sleep Quality: ★☆☆☆☆

Weather: ☀ ☁ ⛅ 🌧 🌦 ❄ Temp: _____

BM Pressure: _____ Allergen Levels: _____

Water: ⊔⊔⊔⊔⊔⊔⊔⊔⊔⊔⊔⊔⊔⊔⊔⊔⊔

Rate Your Pain Level

No Pain (1) (2) (3) (4) (5) (6) (7) (8) (9) (10) Severe pain

Describe your pain / symptoms

	am	pm
	☐	☐
	☐	☐
	☐	☐
	☐	☐
	☐	☐
	☐	☐
	☐	☐

Where does it hurt?

Front   Back

Mood: 😊 😆 😭 😍 😴 😓 😣 😠

Energy Level: (1) (2) (3) (4) (5) (6) (7) (8) (9) (10)

Stress Level: (1) (2) (3) (4) (5) (6) (7) (8) (9) (10)

Mental Clarity: (1) (2) (3) (4) (5) (6) (7) (8) (9) (10)

Feeling Sick?   ☐ Yes ☐ No

☐ Nausea   ☐ Vomiting   ☐ Congestion   ☐ Fever
☐ Diarrhea   ☐ Sore Throat   ☐ Coughing   ☐ Chills

Medications	Time	Dose

Breakfast:

Lunch:

Dinner:

Snacks:

Exercise

☐ None   ☐ Stretching   ☐ Running/Jogging ☐ Yoga
☐ Walking   ☐ Cardio/Weights   ☐

Notes:

Date: _____ Hours of Sleep: _____ Sleep Quality: ★☆☆☆☆

Weather: ☀ ☁ ⛅ 🌧 🌦 ❄ Temp: _____

BM Pressure: _____ Allergen Levels: _____

Water: ⊔⊔⊔⊔⊔⊔⊔⊔⊔⊔⊔⊔⊔⊔⊔⊔⊔⊔

— Rate Your Pain Level —

No Pain ① ② ③ ④ ⑤ ⑥ ⑦ ⑧ ⑨ ⑩ Severe pain

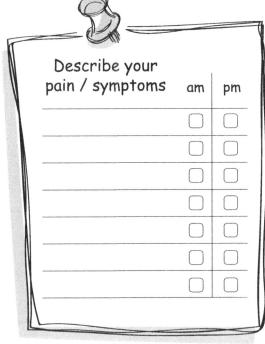

Describe your pain / symptoms

	am	pm
	☐	☐
	☐	☐
	☐	☐
	☐	☐
	☐	☐
	☐	☐
	☐	☐

Where does it hurt?

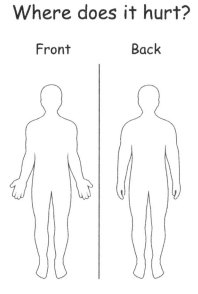

Front   Back

Mood: 😊 😆 😫 😍 😴 😓 😟 😠

Energy Level: ① ② ③ ④ ⑤ ⑥ ⑦ ⑧ ⑨ ⑩

Stress Level: ① ② ③ ④ ⑤ ⑥ ⑦ ⑧ ⑨ ⑩

Mental Clarity: ① ② ③ ④ ⑤ ⑥ ⑦ ⑧ ⑨ ⑩

Feeling Sick? ☐ Yes ☐ No

☐ Nausea   ☐ Vomiting   ☐ Congestion   ☐ Fever

☐ Diarrhea   ☐ Sore Throat   ☐ Coughing   ☐ Chills

Medications	Time	Dose

Breakfast:

Lunch:

Dinner:

Snacks:

Exercise

☐ None   ☐ Stretching   ☐ Running/Jogging ☐ Yoga

☐ Walking   ☐ Cardio/Weights   ☐

Notes:

Date: _____ Hours of Sleep: _____ Sleep Quality: ★☆☆☆☆

Weather: ☀ ☁ ⛅ 🌧 🌦 ❄ Temp: _____

BM Pressure: _____ Allergen Levels: _____

Water: ⊔⊔⊔⊔⊔⊔⊔⊔⊔⊔⊔⊔⊔⊔⊔⊔⊔⊔

--- Rate Your Pain Level ---

No Pain ① ② ③ ④ ⑤ ⑥ ⑦ ⑧ ⑨ ⑩ Severe pain

Describe your pain / symptoms

	am	pm
_____	☐	☐
_____	☐	☐
_____	☐	☐
_____	☐	☐
_____	☐	☐
_____	☐	☐
_____	☐	☐

Where does it hurt?

Front   Back

Mood:	🙂 😝 😣 😍 😴 😓 😧 😠
Energy Level:	① ② ③ ④ ⑤ ⑥ ⑦ ⑧ ⑨ ⑩
Stress Level:	① ② ③ ④ ⑤ ⑥ ⑦ ⑧ ⑨ ⑩
Mental Clarity:	① ② ③ ④ ⑤ ⑥ ⑦ ⑧ ⑨ ⑩

Feeling Sick? ☐ Yes ☐ No

☐ Nausea   ☐ Vomiting   ☐ Congestion   ☐ Fever

☐ Diarrhea ☐ Sore Throat   ☐ Coughing   ☐ Chills

Medications	Time	Dose

Breakfast:

Lunch:

Dinner:

Snacks:

Exercise

☐ None   ☐ Stretching   ☐ Running/Jogging ☐ Yoga

☐ Walking   ☐ Cardio/Weights ☐

Notes:

Date: _____ Hours of Sleep: _____ Sleep Quality: ★☆☆☆☆

Weather: ☀ ☁ ⛅ 🌧 🌦 ❄ Temp: _____

BM Pressure: _____ Allergen Levels: _____

Water: ▢▢▢▢▢▢▢▢▢▢▢▢▢▢▢▢▢▢

——— Rate Your Pain Level ———

No Pain ① ② ③ ④ ⑤ ⑥ ⑦ ⑧ ⑨ ⑩ Severe pain

Describe your pain / symptoms

	am	pm
_____	▢	▢
_____	▢	▢
_____	▢	▢
_____	▢	▢
_____	▢	▢
_____	▢	▢
_____	▢	▢

Where does it hurt?

Front   Back

Mood:	🙂 😆 😭 😍 😴 🤒 😟 😠
Energy Level:	① ② ③ ④ ⑤ ⑥ ⑦ ⑧ ⑨ ⑩
Stress Level:	① ② ③ ④ ⑤ ⑥ ⑦ ⑧ ⑨ ⑩
Mental Clarity:	① ② ③ ④ ⑤ ⑥ ⑦ ⑧ ⑨ ⑩

Feeling Sick? ☐ Yes ☐ No

☐ Nausea   ☐ Vomiting   ☐ Congestion   ☐ Fever
☐ Diarrhea   ☐ Sore Throat   ☐ Coughing   ☐ Chills

Medications	Time	Dose

Breakfast:

Lunch:

Dinner:

Snacks:

Exercise

☐ None   ☐ Stretching   ☐ Running/Jogging ☐ Yoga
☐ Walking   ☐ Cardio/Weights   ☐

Notes:

Date: _____ Hours of Sleep: _____ Sleep Quality: ★☆☆☆☆

Weather: ☀ ☁ ⛅ 🌧 🌦 ❄ Temp: _____

BM Pressure: _____ Allergen Levels: _____

Water: ▢▢▢▢▢▢▢▢▢▢▢▢▢▢▢▢▢▢

Rate Your Pain Level

No Pain ① ② ③ ④ ⑤ ⑥ ⑦ ⑧ ⑨ ⑩ Severe pain

Describe your pain / symptoms

	am	pm
	▢	▢
	▢	▢
	▢	▢
	▢	▢
	▢	▢
	▢	▢
	▢	▢

Where does it hurt?

Front   Back

Mood: 😊 😆 😭 😍 😴 😓 😧 😠

Energy Level: ① ② ③ ④ ⑤ ⑥ ⑦ ⑧ ⑨ ⑩

Stress Level: ① ② ③ ④ ⑤ ⑥ ⑦ ⑧ ⑨ ⑩

Mental Clarity: ① ② ③ ④ ⑤ ⑥ ⑦ ⑧ ⑨ ⑩

Feeling Sick? ☐ Yes ☐ No

☐ Nausea   ☐ Vomiting   ☐ Congestion   ☐ Fever

☐ Diarrhea   ☐ Sore Throat   ☐ Coughing   ☐ Chills

Medications	Time	Dose

Breakfast:

Lunch:

Dinner:

Snacks:

Exercise

☐ None   ☐ Stretching   ☐ Running/Jogging ☐ Yoga

☐ Walking   ☐ Cardio/Weights   ☐

Notes:

Date: _____ Hours of Sleep: _____ Sleep Quality: ★☆☆☆☆

Weather: ☀ ☁ ⛅ 🌧 🌦 ❄ Temp: _____

BM Pressure: _____ Allergen Levels: _____

Water: ⬜⬜⬜⬜⬜⬜⬜⬜⬜⬜⬜⬜⬜⬜⬜⬜⬜⬜

——— Rate Your Pain Level ———

No Pain ① ② ③ ④ ⑤ ⑥ ⑦ ⑧ ⑨ ⑩ Severe pain

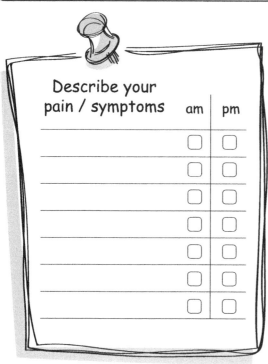

Describe your pain / symptoms

	am	pm
_____	☐	☐
_____	☐	☐
_____	☐	☐
_____	☐	☐
_____	☐	☐
_____	☐	☐
_____	☐	☐

Where does it hurt?

Front   Back

Mood: 🙂 😖 😭 😍 😴 😓 😧 😠

Energy Level: ① ② ③ ④ ⑤ ⑥ ⑦ ⑧ ⑨ ⑩

Stress Level: ① ② ③ ④ ⑤ ⑥ ⑦ ⑧ ⑨ ⑩

Mental Clarity: ① ② ③ ④ ⑤ ⑥ ⑦ ⑧ ⑨ ⑩

Feeling Sick? ☐ Yes ☐ No

☐ Nausea ☐ Vomiting ☐ Congestion ☐ Fever

☐ Diarrhea ☐ Sore Throat ☐ Coughing ☐ Chills

Medications	Time	Dose

Breakfast:

Lunch:

Dinner:

Snacks:

Exercise

☐ None ☐ Stretching ☐ Running/Jogging ☐ Yoga

☐ Walking ☐ Cardio/Weights ☐

Notes:

Date: _____ Hours of Sleep: _____ Sleep Quality: ★☆☆☆☆

Weather: ☀ ☁ ⛅ 🌧 🌦 ❄ Temp: _____

BM Pressure: _____ Allergen Levels: _____

Water: ⊔⊔⊔⊔⊔⊔⊔⊔⊔⊔⊔⊔⊔⊔⊔⊔⊔⊔⊔⊔

Rate Your Pain Level

No Pain ① ② ③ ④ ⑤ ⑥ ⑦ ⑧ ⑨ ⑩ Severe pain

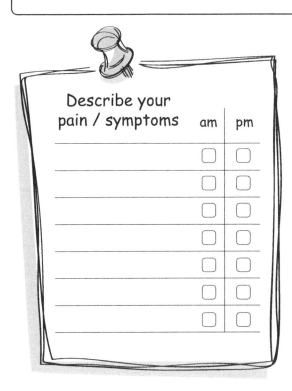

Describe your pain / symptoms

	am	pm
	☐	☐
	☐	☐
	☐	☐
	☐	☐
	☐	☐
	☐	☐
	☐	☐

Where does it hurt?

Front   Back

Mood: 🙂 😆 😭 😍 😴 🥵 😣 😠

Energy Level: ① ② ③ ④ ⑤ ⑥ ⑦ ⑧ ⑨ ⑩

Stress Level: ① ② ③ ④ ⑤ ⑥ ⑦ ⑧ ⑨ ⑩

Mental Clarity: ① ② ③ ④ ⑤ ⑥ ⑦ ⑧ ⑨ ⑩

Feeling Sick? ☐ Yes ☐ No

☐ Nausea   ☐ Vomiting   ☐ Congestion   ☐ Fever

☐ Diarrhea   ☐ Sore Throat   ☐ Coughing   ☐ Chills

Medications	Time	Dose

Breakfast:

Lunch:

Dinner:

Snacks:

Exercise

☐ None   ☐ Stretching   ☐ Running/Jogging ☐ Yoga

☐ Walking   ☐ Cardio/Weights   ☐

Notes:

Date: _____ Hours of Sleep: _____ Sleep Quality: ★☆☆☆☆

Weather: ☀ ☁ ⛅ 🌧 🌦 ❄ Temp: _____

BM Pressure: _____ Allergen Levels: _____

Water: ⊔⊔⊔⊔⊔⊔⊔⊔⊔⊔⊔⊔⊔⊔⊔⊔⊔⊔⊔⊔

Rate Your Pain Level

No Pain ① ② ③ ④ ⑤ ⑥ ⑦ ⑧ ⑨ ⑩ Severe pain

Describe your pain / symptoms

	am	pm
	☐	☐
	☐	☐
	☐	☐
	☐	☐
	☐	☐
	☐	☐
	☐	☐

Where does it hurt?

Front   Back

Mood: 🙂 😣 😭 😍 😴 😓 😟 😠

Energy Level: ① ② ③ ④ ⑤ ⑥ ⑦ ⑧ ⑨ ⑩

Stress Level: ① ② ③ ④ ⑤ ⑥ ⑦ ⑧ ⑨ ⑩

Mental Clarity: ① ② ③ ④ ⑤ ⑥ ⑦ ⑧ ⑨ ⑩

Feeling Sick? ☐ Yes ☐ No

☐ Nausea   ☐ Vomiting   ☐ Congestion   ☐ Fever

☐ Diarrhea   ☐ Sore Throat   ☐ Coughing   ☐ Chills

Medications	Time	Dose

Breakfast:

Lunch:

Dinner:

Snacks:

Exercise

☐ None   ☐ Stretching   ☐ Running/Jogging ☐ Yoga

☐ Walking   ☐ Cardio/Weights   ☐

Notes:

Date: _____ Hours of Sleep: _____ Sleep Quality: ⭐️☆☆☆☆

Weather: ☀️ ☁️ ⛅️ 🌧️ 🌦️ ❄️ Temp: _____

BM Pressure: _____ Allergen Levels: _____

Water: ⬜️⬜️⬜️⬜️⬜️⬜️⬜️⬜️⬜️⬜️⬜️⬜️⬜️⬜️⬜️⬜️⬜️

Rate Your Pain Level

No Pain ① ② ③ ④ ⑤ ⑥ ⑦ ⑧ ⑨ ⑩ Severe pain

Describe your pain / symptoms

	am	pm
_____	☐	☐
_____	☐	☐
_____	☐	☐
_____	☐	☐
_____	☐	☐
_____	☐	☐
_____	☐	☐

Where does it hurt?

Front   Back

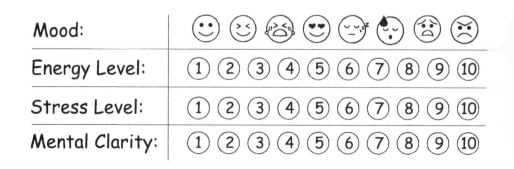

Mood:	🙂 😆 😭 😍 😴 😰 😧 😠
Energy Level:	① ② ③ ④ ⑤ ⑥ ⑦ ⑧ ⑨ ⑩
Stress Level:	① ② ③ ④ ⑤ ⑥ ⑦ ⑧ ⑨ ⑩
Mental Clarity:	① ② ③ ④ ⑤ ⑥ ⑦ ⑧ ⑨ ⑩

Feeling Sick? ☐ Yes ☐ No

☐ Nausea ☐ Vomiting ☐ Congestion ☐ Fever

☐ Diarrhea ☐ Sore Throat ☐ Coughing ☐ Chills

Medications	Time	Dose

Breakfast:

Lunch:

Dinner:

Snacks:

Exercise

☐ None ☐ Stretching ☐ Running/Jogging ☐ Yoga

☐ Walking ☐ Cardio/Weights ☐

Notes:

Date: _____ Hours of Sleep: _____ Sleep Quality: ★☆☆☆☆

Weather: ☀ ☁ ⛅ 🌧 🌦 ❄ Temp: _____

BM Pressure: _____ Allergen Levels: _____

Water: ▢▢▢▢▢▢▢▢▢▢▢▢▢▢▢▢▢

Rate Your Pain Level

No Pain ① ② ③ ④ ⑤ ⑥ ⑦ ⑧ ⑨ ⑩ Severe pain

Describe your pain / symptoms	am	pm
	▢	▢
	▢	▢
	▢	▢
	▢	▢
	▢	▢
	▢	▢
	▢	▢

Where does it hurt?

Front   Back

Mood: 😊 😝 😭 😍 😴 😓 😣 😠

Energy Level: ① ② ③ ④ ⑤ ⑥ ⑦ ⑧ ⑨ ⑩

Stress Level: ① ② ③ ④ ⑤ ⑥ ⑦ ⑧ ⑨ ⑩

Mental Clarity: ① ② ③ ④ ⑤ ⑥ ⑦ ⑧ ⑨ ⑩

Feeling Sick? ☐ Yes ☐ No

☐ Nausea ☐ Vomiting ☐ Congestion ☐ Fever
☐ Diarrhea ☐ Sore Throat ☐ Coughing ☐ Chills

Medications	Time	Dose

Breakfast:

Lunch:

Dinner:

Snacks:

Exercise

☐ None ☐ Stretching ☐ Running/Jogging ☐ Yoga
☐ Walking ☐ Cardio/Weights ☐

Notes:

Date: _____ Hours of Sleep: _____ Sleep Quality: ★☆☆☆☆

Weather: ☀ ☁ ⛅ 🌧 🌦 ❄ Temp: _____

BM Pressure: _____ Allergen Levels: _____

Water: ▢▢▢▢▢▢▢▢▢▢▢▢▢▢▢▢

Rate Your Pain Level

No Pain ① ② ③ ④ ⑤ ⑥ ⑦ ⑧ ⑨ ⑩ Severe pain

Describe your pain / symptoms

	am	pm
_____	▢	▢
_____	▢	▢
_____	▢	▢
_____	▢	▢
_____	▢	▢
_____	▢	▢
_____	▢	▢

Where does it hurt?

Front   Back

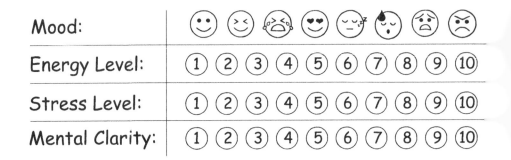

Mood:	😊 😖 😫 😍 😴 😓 😟 😠
Energy Level:	① ② ③ ④ ⑤ ⑥ ⑦ ⑧ ⑨ ⑩
Stress Level:	① ② ③ ④ ⑤ ⑥ ⑦ ⑧ ⑨ ⑩
Mental Clarity:	① ② ③ ④ ⑤ ⑥ ⑦ ⑧ ⑨ ⑩

Feeling Sick? ☐ Yes ☐ No

☐ Nausea   ☐ Vomiting   ☐ Congestion   ☐ Fever
☐ Diarrhea   ☐ Sore Throat   ☐ Coughing   ☐ Chills

Medications	Time	Dose

Breakfast:

Lunch:

Dinner:

Snacks:

Exercise

☐ None   ☐ Stretching   ☐ Running/Jogging ☐ Yoga
☐ Walking ☐ Cardio/Weights   ☐

Notes:

Date: _____ Hours of Sleep: _____ Sleep Quality: ★☆☆☆☆

Weather: ☀ ☁ ⛅ 🌧 🌦 ❄ Temp: _____

BM Pressure: _____ Allergen Levels: _____

Water: ⊔⊔⊔⊔⊔⊔⊔⊔⊔⊔⊔⊔⊔⊔⊔⊔⊔⊔⊔⊔

Rate Your Pain Level

No Pain ① ② ③ ④ ⑤ ⑥ ⑦ ⑧ ⑨ ⑩ Severe pain

Describe your pain / symptoms

	am	pm
_____	☐	☐
_____	☐	☐
_____	☐	☐
_____	☐	☐
_____	☐	☐
_____	☐	☐
_____	☐	☐

Where does it hurt?

Front   Back

Mood: 🙂 😆 😭 😍 😴 😓 😣 😠

Energy Level: ① ② ③ ④ ⑤ ⑥ ⑦ ⑧ ⑨ ⑩

Stress Level: ① ② ③ ④ ⑤ ⑥ ⑦ ⑧ ⑨ ⑩

Mental Clarity: ① ② ③ ④ ⑤ ⑥ ⑦ ⑧ ⑨ ⑩

Feeling Sick? ☐ Yes ☐ No

☐ Nausea ☐ Vomiting ☐ Congestion ☐ Fever
☐ Diarrhea ☐ Sore Throat ☐ Coughing ☐ Chills

Medications	Time	Dose

Breakfast:

Lunch:

Dinner:

Snacks:

Exercise

☐ None ☐ Stretching ☐ Running/Jogging ☐ Yoga
☐ Walking ☐ Cardio/Weights ☐

Notes:

Date: _____ Hours of Sleep: _____ Sleep Quality: ★☆☆☆☆

Weather: ☀ ☁ ⛅ 🌧 🌦 ❄ Temp: _____

BM Pressure: _____ Allergen Levels: _____

Water: ⊔⊔⊔⊔⊔⊔⊔⊔⊔⊔⊔⊔⊔⊔⊔⊔⊔⊔

Rate Your Pain Level

No Pain ① ② ③ ④ ⑤ ⑥ ⑦ ⑧ ⑨ ⑩ Severe pain

Describe your pain / symptoms

	am	pm
_____	☐	☐
_____	☐	☐
_____	☐	☐
_____	☐	☐
_____	☐	☐
_____	☐	☐
_____	☐	☐

Where does it hurt?

Front   Back

Mood:	😊 😆 😭 😍 😌 😓 😣 😠
Energy Level:	① ② ③ ④ ⑤ ⑥ ⑦ ⑧ ⑨ ⑩
Stress Level:	① ② ③ ④ ⑤ ⑥ ⑦ ⑧ ⑨ ⑩
Mental Clarity:	① ② ③ ④ ⑤ ⑥ ⑦ ⑧ ⑨ ⑩

Feeling Sick? ☐ Yes ☐ No

☐ Nausea   ☐ Vomiting   ☐ Congestion   ☐ Fever

☐ Diarrhea ☐ Sore Throat ☐ Coughing   ☐ Chills

Medications	Time	Dose

Breakfast:

Lunch:

Dinner:

Snacks:

Exercise

☐ None   ☐ Stretching   ☐ Running/Jogging ☐ Yoga

☐ Walking   ☐ Cardio/Weights ☐

Notes:

Date: _____ Hours of Sleep: _____ Sleep Quality: ★☆☆☆☆

Weather: ☀ ☁ ⛅ 🌧 🌦 ❄ Temp: _____

BM Pressure: _____ Allergen Levels: _____

Water: ▢▢▢▢▢▢▢▢▢▢▢▢▢▢▢▢▢▢▢▢

— Rate Your Pain Level —

No Pain ① ② ③ ④ ⑤ ⑥ ⑦ ⑧ ⑨ ⑩ Severe pain

Describe your pain / symptoms

	am	pm
	▢	▢
	▢	▢
	▢	▢
	▢	▢
	▢	▢
	▢	▢
	▢	▢

Where does it hurt?

Front   Back

Mood:	🙂 😆 😭 😍 😴 😓 😟 😠
Energy Level:	① ② ③ ④ ⑤ ⑥ ⑦ ⑧ ⑨ ⑩
Stress Level:	① ② ③ ④ ⑤ ⑥ ⑦ ⑧ ⑨ ⑩
Mental Clarity:	① ② ③ ④ ⑤ ⑥ ⑦ ⑧ ⑨ ⑩

Feeling Sick? ☐ Yes ☐ No

☐ Nausea   ☐ Vomiting   ☐ Congestion   ☐ Fever

☐ Diarrhea   ☐ Sore Throat   ☐ Coughing   ☐ Chills

Medications	Time	Dose

Breakfast:

Lunch:

Dinner:

Snacks:

Exercise

☐ None   ☐ Stretching   ☐ Running/Jogging ☐ Yoga

☐ Walking   ☐ Cardio/Weights   ☐

Notes:

Date: _____ Hours of Sleep: _____ Sleep Quality: ★☆☆☆☆

Weather: ☀ ☁ ⛅ 🌧 🌦 ❄ Temp: _____

BM Pressure: _____ Allergen Levels: _____

Water: ⊔⊔⊔⊔⊔⊔⊔⊔⊔⊔⊔⊔⊔⊔⊔⊔⊔⊔

Rate Your Pain Level

No Pain ① ② ③ ④ ⑤ ⑥ ⑦ ⑧ ⑨ ⑩ Severe pain

Describe your pain / symptoms

	am	pm
_____	☐	☐
_____	☐	☐
_____	☐	☐
_____	☐	☐
_____	☐	☐
_____	☐	☐
_____	☐	☐

Where does it hurt?

Front   Back

Mood: 😊 😣 😖 😍 😴 😓 😧 😠

Energy Level: ① ② ③ ④ ⑤ ⑥ ⑦ ⑧ ⑨ ⑩

Stress Level: ① ② ③ ④ ⑤ ⑥ ⑦ ⑧ ⑨ ⑩

Mental Clarity: ① ② ③ ④ ⑤ ⑥ ⑦ ⑧ ⑨ ⑩

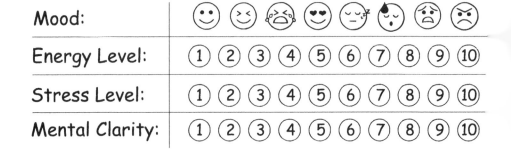

Feeling Sick? ☐ Yes ☐ No

☐ Nausea   ☐ Vomiting   ☐ Congestion   ☐ Fever

☐ Diarrhea   ☐ Sore Throat   ☐ Coughing   ☐ Chills

Medications	Time	Dose

Breakfast:

Lunch:

Dinner:

Snacks:

Exercise

☐ None   ☐ Stretching   ☐ Running/Jogging ☐ Yoga

☐ Walking   ☐ Cardio/Weights   ☐

Notes:

Date: _____ Hours of Sleep: _____ Sleep Quality: ★☆☆☆☆

Weather: ☀ ☁ ⛅ 🌧 🌦 ❄ Temp: _____

BM Pressure: _____ Allergen Levels: _____

Water: ▽▽▽▽▽▽▽▽▽▽▽▽▽▽▽▽▽▽

Rate Your Pain Level

No Pain ① ② ③ ④ ⑤ ⑥ ⑦ ⑧ ⑨ ⑩ Severe pain

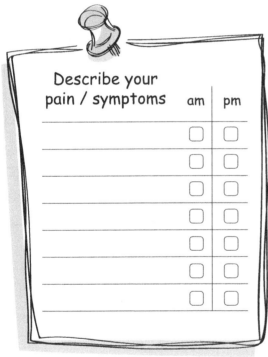

Describe your pain / symptoms

	am	pm
	☐	☐
	☐	☐
	☐	☐
	☐	☐
	☐	☐
	☐	☐
	☐	☐

Where does it hurt?

Front   Back

Mood:	🙂 😖 😫 😍 😴 😓 😣 😠
Energy Level:	① ② ③ ④ ⑤ ⑥ ⑦ ⑧ ⑨ ⑩
Stress Level:	① ② ③ ④ ⑤ ⑥ ⑦ ⑧ ⑨ ⑩
Mental Clarity:	① ② ③ ④ ⑤ ⑥ ⑦ ⑧ ⑨ ⑩

Feeling Sick? ☐ Yes ☐ No

☐ Nausea ☐ Vomiting ☐ Congestion ☐ Fever

☐ Diarrhea ☐ Sore Throat ☐ Coughing ☐ Chills

Medications	Time	Dose

Breakfast:

Lunch:

Dinner:

Snacks:

Exercise

☐ None ☐ Stretching ☐ Running/Jogging ☐ Yoga

☐ Walking ☐ Cardio/Weights ☐

Notes:

Date: _____ Hours of Sleep: _____ Sleep Quality: ★☆☆☆☆

Weather: ☀ ☁ ⛅ 🌧 🌦 ❄ Temp: _____

BM Pressure: _____ Allergen Levels: _____

Water: ⊔⊔⊔⊔⊔⊔⊔⊔⊔⊔⊔⊔⊔⊔⊔⊔⊔⊔⊔⊔

Rate Your Pain Level

No Pain ① ② ③ ④ ⑤ ⑥ ⑦ ⑧ ⑨ ⑩ Severe pain

Describe your pain / symptoms

	am	pm
_____	☐	☐
_____	☐	☐
_____	☐	☐
_____	☐	☐
_____	☐	☐
_____	☐	☐
_____	☐	☐

Where does it hurt?

Front   Back

Mood: 😊 😆 😫 😍 😴 😓 😩 😠

Energy Level: ① ② ③ ④ ⑤ ⑥ ⑦ ⑧ ⑨ ⑩

Stress Level: ① ② ③ ④ ⑤ ⑥ ⑦ ⑧ ⑨ ⑩

Mental Clarity: ① ② ③ ④ ⑤ ⑥ ⑦ ⑧ ⑨ ⑩

Feeling Sick? ☐ Yes ☐ No

☐ Nausea   ☐ Vomiting   ☐ Congestion   ☐ Fever

☐ Diarrhea ☐ Sore Throat ☐ Coughing   ☐ Chills

Medications	Time	Dose

Breakfast:

Lunch:

Dinner:

Snacks:

Exercise

☐ None   ☐ Stretching   ☐ Running/Jogging ☐ Yoga

☐ Walking ☐ Cardio/Weights ☐

Notes:

Date: _____ Hours of Sleep: _____ Sleep Quality: ★☆☆☆☆

Weather: ☀ ☁ ⛅ 🌧 🌦 ❄ Temp: _____

BM Pressure: _____ Allergen Levels: _____

Water: ⊔⊔⊔⊔⊔⊔⊔⊔⊔⊔⊔⊔⊔⊔⊔⊔⊔⊔

Rate Your Pain Level

No Pain ① ② ③ ④ ⑤ ⑥ ⑦ ⑧ ⑨ ⑩ Severe pain

Describe your pain / symptoms

	am	pm
_____	☐	☐
_____	☐	☐
_____	☐	☐
_____	☐	☐
_____	☐	☐
_____	☐	☐
_____	☐	☐

Where does it hurt?

Front   Back

Mood:	🙂 😆 😫 😍 😴 😓 😖 😠
Energy Level:	① ② ③ ④ ⑤ ⑥ ⑦ ⑧ ⑨ ⑩
Stress Level:	① ② ③ ④ ⑤ ⑥ ⑦ ⑧ ⑨ ⑩
Mental Clarity:	① ② ③ ④ ⑤ ⑥ ⑦ ⑧ ⑨ ⑩

Feeling Sick? ☐ Yes ☐ No

☐ Nausea   ☐ Vomiting   ☐ Congestion   ☐ Fever

☐ Diarrhea ☐ Sore Throat   ☐ Coughing   ☐ Chills

Medications	Time	Dose

Breakfast:

Lunch:

Dinner:

Snacks:

Exercise

☐ None   ☐ Stretching   ☐ Running/Jogging ☐ Yoga

☐ Walking ☐ Cardio/Weights   ☐

Notes:

Date: _____ Hours of Sleep: _____ Sleep Quality: ★☆☆☆☆

Weather: ☀ ☁ ⛅ 🌧 🌦 ❄ Temp: _____

BM Pressure: _____ Allergen Levels: _____

Water: ⬜⬜⬜⬜⬜⬜⬜⬜⬜⬜⬜⬜⬜⬜⬜⬜⬜⬜

Rate Your Pain Level

No Pain ① ② ③ ④ ⑤ ⑥ ⑦ ⑧ ⑨ ⑩ Severe pain

Describe your pain / symptoms

	am	pm
_____	☐	☐
_____	☐	☐
_____	☐	☐
_____	☐	☐
_____	☐	☐
_____	☐	☐
_____	☐	☐

Where does it hurt?

Front   Back

Mood:	🙂 😝 😭 😍 😴 🥵 😣 😠
Energy Level:	① ② ③ ④ ⑤ ⑥ ⑦ ⑧ ⑨ ⑩
Stress Level:	① ② ③ ④ ⑤ ⑥ ⑦ ⑧ ⑨ ⑩
Mental Clarity:	① ② ③ ④ ⑤ ⑥ ⑦ ⑧ ⑨ ⑩

Feeling Sick? ☐ Yes ☐ No

☐ Nausea   ☐ Vomiting   ☐ Congestion   ☐ Fever

☐ Diarrhea   ☐ Sore Throat   ☐ Coughing   ☐ Chills

Medications	Time	Dose

Breakfast:

Lunch:

Dinner:

Snacks:

Exercise

☐ None   ☐ Stretching   ☐ Running/Jogging ☐ Yoga

☐ Walking   ☐ Cardio/Weights   ☐

Notes:

Date: _____ Hours of Sleep: _____ Sleep Quality: ★☆☆☆☆

Weather: ☀ ☁ ⛅ ☁ ⛅ ❄ Temp: _____

BM Pressure: _____ Allergen Levels: _____

Water: ▢▢▢▢▢▢▢▢▢▢▢▢▢▢▢▢▢

── Rate Your Pain Level ──

No Pain ① ② ③ ④ ⑤ ⑥ ⑦ ⑧ ⑨ ⑩ Severe pain

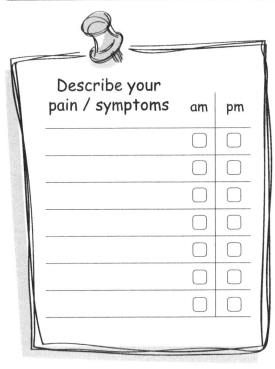

Describe your pain / symptoms

	am	pm
	▢	▢
	▢	▢
	▢	▢
	▢	▢
	▢	▢
	▢	▢
	▢	▢

Where does it hurt?

Front   Back

Mood: 🙂 😆 😫 😍 😴 😓 😧 😠

Energy Level: ① ② ③ ④ ⑤ ⑥ ⑦ ⑧ ⑨ ⑩

Stress Level: ① ② ③ ④ ⑤ ⑥ ⑦ ⑧ ⑨ ⑩

Mental Clarity: ① ② ③ ④ ⑤ ⑥ ⑦ ⑧ ⑨ ⑩

Feeling Sick?   ☐ Yes ☐ No

☐ Nausea   ☐ Vomiting   ☐ Congestion   ☐ Fever

☐ Diarrhea   ☐ Sore Throat   ☐ Coughing   ☐ Chills

Medications	Time	Dose

Breakfast:

Lunch:

Dinner:

Snacks:

Exercise

☐ None   ☐ Stretching   ☐ Running/Jogging ☐ Yoga

☐ Walking   ☐ Cardio/Weights   ☐

Notes:

Date: _____ Hours of Sleep: _____ Sleep Quality: ★☆☆☆☆

Weather: ☀ ☁ ⛅ 🌧 🌦 ❄ Temp: _____

BM Pressure: _____ Allergen Levels: _____

Water: ⬜⬜⬜⬜⬜⬜⬜⬜⬜⬜⬜⬜⬜⬜⬜⬜⬜⬜

Rate Your Pain Level

No Pain ① ② ③ ④ ⑤ ⑥ ⑦ ⑧ ⑨ ⑩ Severe pain

Describe your pain / symptoms

	am	pm
_____	☐	☐
_____	☐	☐
_____	☐	☐
_____	☐	☐
_____	☐	☐
_____	☐	☐
_____	☐	☐

Where does it hurt?

Front   Back

Mood: 🙂 😆 😭 😍 😌 😓 😟 😠

Energy Level: ① ② ③ ④ ⑤ ⑥ ⑦ ⑧ ⑨ ⑩

Stress Level: ① ② ③ ④ ⑤ ⑥ ⑦ ⑧ ⑨ ⑩

Mental Clarity: ① ② ③ ④ ⑤ ⑥ ⑦ ⑧ ⑨ ⑩

Feeling Sick? ☐ Yes ☐ No

☐ Nausea   ☐ Vomiting   ☐ Congestion   ☐ Fever

☐ Diarrhea   ☐ Sore Throat   ☐ Coughing   ☐ Chills

Medications	Time	Dose

Breakfast:

Lunch:

Dinner:

Snacks:

Exercise

☐ None   ☐ Stretching   ☐ Running/Jogging ☐ Yoga

☐ Walking   ☐ Cardio/Weights   ☐

Notes:

Date: _____ Hours of Sleep: _____ Sleep Quality: ★☆☆☆☆☆

Weather: ☀ ☁ ⛅ 🌧 🌦 ❄ Temp: _____

BM Pressure: _____ Allergen Levels: _____

Water: ⊔⊔⊔⊔⊔⊔⊔⊔⊔⊔⊔⊔⊔⊔⊔⊔⊔⊔

Rate Your Pain Level

No Pain ① ② ③ ④ ⑤ ⑥ ⑦ ⑧ ⑨ ⑩ Severe pain

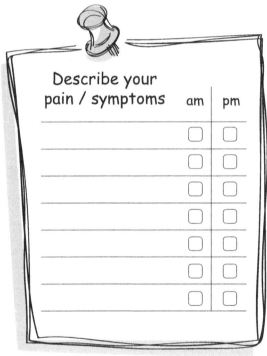

Describe your pain / symptoms | am | pm

Where does it hurt?

Front   Back

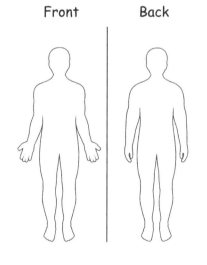

Mood:	🙂 😣 😭 😍 😴 🥵 😩 😠
Energy Level:	① ② ③ ④ ⑤ ⑥ ⑦ ⑧ ⑨ ⑩
Stress Level:	① ② ③ ④ ⑤ ⑥ ⑦ ⑧ ⑨ ⑩
Mental Clarity:	① ② ③ ④ ⑤ ⑥ ⑦ ⑧ ⑨ ⑩

Feeling Sick? ☐ Yes ☐ No

☐ Nausea   ☐ Vomiting   ☐ Congestion   ☐ Fever
☐ Diarrhea ☐ Sore Throat ☐ Coughing   ☐ Chills

Medications	Time	Dose

Breakfast:

Lunch:

Dinner:

Snacks:

Exercise

☐ None   ☐ Stretching   ☐ Running/Jogging ☐ Yoga
☐ Walking ☐ Cardio/Weights ☐

Notes:

Date: _____ Hours of Sleep: _____ Sleep Quality: ★☆☆☆☆

Weather: ☀ ☁ ⛅ 🌧 🌦 ❄ Temp: _____

BM Pressure: _____ Allergen Levels: _____

Water: ▢▢▢▢▢▢▢▢▢▢▢▢▢▢▢▢▢▢▢▢

— Rate Your Pain Level —

No Pain ① ② ③ ④ ⑤ ⑥ ⑦ ⑧ ⑨ ⑩ Severe pain

Describe your pain / symptoms

	am	pm
_____	☐	☐
_____	☐	☐
_____	☐	☐
_____	☐	☐
_____	☐	☐
_____	☐	☐
_____	☐	☐

Where does it hurt?

Front   Back

Mood: 🙂 😆 😣 😍 😴 😓 😧 😠

Energy Level: ① ② ③ ④ ⑤ ⑥ ⑦ ⑧ ⑨ ⑩

Stress Level: ① ② ③ ④ ⑤ ⑥ ⑦ ⑧ ⑨ ⑩

Mental Clarity: ① ② ③ ④ ⑤ ⑥ ⑦ ⑧ ⑨ ⑩

Feeling Sick? ☐ Yes ☐ No

☐ Nausea ☐ Vomiting ☐ Congestion ☐ Fever
☐ Diarrhea ☐ Sore Throat ☐ Coughing ☐ Chills

Medications	Time	Dose

Breakfast:

Lunch:

Dinner:

Snacks:

Exercise

☐ None ☐ Stretching ☐ Running/Jogging ☐ Yoga
☐ Walking ☐ Cardio/Weights ☐

Notes:

Date: _____ Hours of Sleep: _____ Sleep Quality: ★☆☆☆☆

Weather: ☀ ☁ ⛅ 🌧 🌦 ❄ Temp: _____

BM Pressure: _____ Allergen Levels: _____

Water: ⊔⊔⊔⊔⊔⊔⊔⊔⊔⊔⊔⊔⊔⊔⊔⊔⊔⊔⊔⊔

Rate Your Pain Level

No Pain (1) (2) (3) (4) (5) (6) (7) (8) (9) (10) Severe pain

Describe your pain / symptoms

	am	pm
	☐	☐
	☐	☐
	☐	☐
	☐	☐
	☐	☐
	☐	☐
	☐	☐

Where does it hurt?

Front   Back

Mood: 🙂 😣 😭 😍 😌 😓 😖 😠

Energy Level: (1) (2) (3) (4) (5) (6) (7) (8) (9) (10)

Stress Level: (1) (2) (3) (4) (5) (6) (7) (8) (9) (10)

Mental Clarity: (1) (2) (3) (4) (5) (6) (7) (8) (9) (10)

Feeling Sick? ☐ Yes ☐ No

☐ Nausea   ☐ Vomiting   ☐ Congestion   ☐ Fever

☐ Diarrhea   ☐ Sore Throat   ☐ Coughing   ☐ Chills

Medications	Time	Dose

Breakfast:

Lunch:

Dinner:

Snacks:

Exercise

☐ None   ☐ Stretching   ☐ Running/Jogging ☐ Yoga

☐ Walking   ☐ Cardio/Weights   ☐

Notes:

Date: _____ Hours of Sleep: _____ Sleep Quality: ★☆☆☆☆

Weather: ☀ ☁ ⛅ 🌧 🌦 ❄ Temp: _____

BM Pressure: _____ Allergen Levels: _____

Water: 🥛🥛🥛🥛🥛🥛🥛🥛🥛🥛🥛🥛🥛🥛🥛🥛🥛🥛

Rate Your Pain Level

No Pain ① ② ③ ④ ⑤ ⑥ ⑦ ⑧ ⑨ ⑩ Severe pain

Describe your pain / symptoms

	am	pm
_____	☐	☐
_____	☐	☐
_____	☐	☐
_____	☐	☐
_____	☐	☐
_____	☐	☐
_____	☐	☐

Where does it hurt?

Front   Back

Mood: 🙂 😆 😭 😍 😴 😓 😩 😠

Energy Level: ① ② ③ ④ ⑤ ⑥ ⑦ ⑧ ⑨ ⑩

Stress Level: ① ② ③ ④ ⑤ ⑥ ⑦ ⑧ ⑨ ⑩

Mental Clarity: ① ② ③ ④ ⑤ ⑥ ⑦ ⑧ ⑨ ⑩

Feeling Sick?　☐ Yes ☐ No

☐ Nausea　☐ Vomiting　☐ Congestion　☐ Fever

☐ Diarrhea　☐ Sore Throat　☐ Coughing　☐ Chills

Medications	Time	Dose

Breakfast:

Lunch:

Dinner:

Snacks:

Exercise

☐ None　☐ Stretching　☐ Running/Jogging ☐ Yoga

☐ Walking　☐ Cardio/Weights　☐

Notes:

Date: _____ Hours of Sleep: _____ Sleep Quality: ★☆☆☆☆

Weather: ☀ ☁ ⛅ 🌧 🌦 ❄ Temp: _____

BM Pressure: _____ Allergen Levels: _____

Water: ⊔⊔⊔⊔⊔⊔⊔⊔⊔⊔⊔⊔⊔⊔⊔⊔⊔⊔⊔⊔

Rate Your Pain Level

No Pain ① ② ③ ④ ⑤ ⑥ ⑦ ⑧ ⑨ ⑩ Severe pain

Describe your pain / symptoms

	am	pm
	☐	☐
	☐	☐
	☐	☐
	☐	☐
	☐	☐
	☐	☐
	☐	☐

Where does it hurt?

Front   Back

Mood:	😊 😆 😭 😍 😌 😓 😧 😠
Energy Level:	① ② ③ ④ ⑤ ⑥ ⑦ ⑧ ⑨ ⑩
Stress Level:	① ② ③ ④ ⑤ ⑥ ⑦ ⑧ ⑨ ⑩
Mental Clarity:	① ② ③ ④ ⑤ ⑥ ⑦ ⑧ ⑨ ⑩

Feeling Sick? ☐ Yes ☐ No

☐ Nausea   ☐ Vomiting   ☐ Congestion   ☐ Fever

☐ Diarrhea ☐ Sore Throat ☐ Coughing   ☐ Chills

Medications	Time	Dose

Breakfast:

Lunch:

Dinner:

Snacks:

Exercise

☐ None   ☐ Stretching   ☐ Running/Jogging ☐ Yoga

☐ Walking ☐ Cardio/Weights ☐

Notes:

Date: _____ Hours of Sleep: _____ Sleep Quality: ★☆☆☆☆

Weather: ☀ ☁ ⛅ 🌧 🌦 ❄ Temp: _____

BM Pressure: _____ Allergen Levels: _____

Water: ▢▢▢▢▢▢▢▢▢▢▢▢▢▢▢▢

Rate Your Pain Level

No Pain ① ② ③ ④ ⑤ ⑥ ⑦ ⑧ ⑨ ⑩ Severe pain

Describe your pain / symptoms

	am	pm
_____	▢	▢
_____	▢	▢
_____	▢	▢
_____	▢	▢
_____	▢	▢
_____	▢	▢
_____	▢	▢

Where does it hurt?

Front   Back

Mood: 🙂 😆 😭 😍 😴 😓 😟 😠

Energy Level: ① ② ③ ④ ⑤ ⑥ ⑦ ⑧ ⑨ ⑩

Stress Level: ① ② ③ ④ ⑤ ⑥ ⑦ ⑧ ⑨ ⑩

Mental Clarity: ① ② ③ ④ ⑤ ⑥ ⑦ ⑧ ⑨ ⑩

Feeling Sick? ☐ Yes ☐ No

☐ Nausea   ☐ Vomiting   ☐ Congestion   ☐ Fever

☐ Diarrhea   ☐ Sore Throat   ☐ Coughing   ☐ Chills

Medications	Time	Dose

Breakfast:

Lunch:

Dinner:

Snacks:

Exercise

☐ None   ☐ Stretching   ☐ Running/Jogging ☐ Yoga

☐ Walking   ☐ Cardio/Weights   ☐

Notes:

Date: _____ Hours of Sleep: _____ Sleep Quality: ★☆☆☆☆☆

Weather: ☀ ☁ ⛅ 🌧 🌦 ❄ Temp: _____

BM Pressure: _____ Allergen Levels: _____

Water: ▯▯▯▯▯▯▯▯▯▯▯▯▯▯▯▯▯

Rate Your Pain Level

No Pain ① ② ③ ④ ⑤ ⑥ ⑦ ⑧ ⑨ ⑩ Severe pain

Describe your pain / symptoms

	am	pm
	☐	☐
	☐	☐
	☐	☐
	☐	☐
	☐	☐
	☐	☐
	☐	☐

Where does it hurt?

Front   Back

Mood: 🙂 😣 😭 😍 😴 😓 😖 😠

Energy Level: ① ② ③ ④ ⑤ ⑥ ⑦ ⑧ ⑨ ⑩

Stress Level: ① ② ③ ④ ⑤ ⑥ ⑦ ⑧ ⑨ ⑩

Mental Clarity: ① ② ③ ④ ⑤ ⑥ ⑦ ⑧ ⑨ ⑩

Feeling Sick? ☐ Yes ☐ No

☐ Nausea   ☐ Vomiting   ☐ Congestion   ☐ Fever

☐ Diarrhea ☐ Sore Throat ☐ Coughing   ☐ Chills

Medications	Time	Dose

Breakfast:

Lunch:

Dinner:

Snacks:

Exercise

☐ None   ☐ Stretching   ☐ Running/Jogging ☐ Yoga

☐ Walking ☐ Cardio/Weights ☐

Notes:

Date: _____ Hours of Sleep: _____ Sleep Quality: ⭐☆☆☆☆

Weather: ☀ ☁ ⛅ 🌧 🌦 ❄ Temp: _____

BM Pressure: _____ Allergen Levels: _____

Water: ⊔⊔⊔⊔⊔⊔⊔⊔⊔⊔⊔⊔⊔⊔⊔⊔⊔⊔⊔⊔

Rate Your Pain Level

No Pain ① ② ③ ④ ⑤ ⑥ ⑦ ⑧ ⑨ ⑩ Severe pain

Describe your pain / symptoms

	am	pm
_____	☐	☐
_____	☐	☐
_____	☐	☐
_____	☐	☐
_____	☐	☐
_____	☐	☐
_____	☐	☐

Where does it hurt?

Front   Back

Mood: 🙂 😣 😭 😍 😴 😓 😧 😠

Energy Level: ① ② ③ ④ ⑤ ⑥ ⑦ ⑧ ⑨ ⑩

Stress Level: ① ② ③ ④ ⑤ ⑥ ⑦ ⑧ ⑨ ⑩

Mental Clarity: ① ② ③ ④ ⑤ ⑥ ⑦ ⑧ ⑨ ⑩

Feeling Sick? ☐ Yes ☐ No

☐ Nausea   ☐ Vomiting   ☐ Congestion   ☐ Fever
☐ Diarrhea   ☐ Sore Throat   ☐ Coughing   ☐ Chills

Medications	Time	Dose

Breakfast:

Lunch:

Dinner:

Snacks:

Exercise

☐ None   ☐ Stretching   ☐ Running/Jogging ☐ Yoga
☐ Walking ☐ Cardio/Weights ☐

Notes:

Date: _____ Hours of Sleep: _____ Sleep Quality: ★☆☆☆☆

Weather: ☀ ☁ ⛅ 🌧 🌦 ❄ Temp: _____

BM Pressure: _____ Allergen Levels: _____

Water: 🥛🥛🥛🥛🥛🥛🥛🥛🥛🥛🥛🥛🥛🥛🥛🥛🥛

Rate Your Pain Level

No Pain (1) (2) (3) (4) (5) (6) (7) (8) (9) (10) Severe pain

Describe your pain / symptoms

	am	pm
_____	☐	☐
_____	☐	☐
_____	☐	☐
_____	☐	☐
_____	☐	☐
_____	☐	☐
_____	☐	☐

Where does it hurt?

Front   Back

Mood:	🙂 😖 😭 😍 😴 😰 😧 😠
Energy Level:	(1) (2) (3) (4) (5) (6) (7) (8) (9) (10)
Stress Level:	(1) (2) (3) (4) (5) (6) (7) (8) (9) (10)
Mental Clarity:	(1) (2) (3) (4) (5) (6) (7) (8) (9) (10)

Feeling Sick? ☐ Yes ☐ No

☐ Nausea ☐ Vomiting ☐ Congestion ☐ Fever
☐ Diarrhea ☐ Sore Throat ☐ Coughing ☐ Chills

Medications	Time	Dose

Breakfast:

Lunch:

Dinner:

Snacks:

Exercise

☐ None ☐ Stretching ☐ Running/Jogging ☐ Yoga
☐ Walking ☐ Cardio/Weights ☐

Notes:

Date: _____ Hours of Sleep: _____ Sleep Quality: ★☆☆☆☆

Weather: ☀ ☁ ⛅ 🌧 🌦 ❄ Temp: _____

BM Pressure: _____ Allergen Levels: _____

Water: ⊔⊔⊔⊔⊔⊔⊔⊔⊔⊔⊔⊔⊔⊔⊔⊔⊔⊔

Rate Your Pain Level

No Pain ① ② ③ ④ ⑤ ⑥ ⑦ ⑧ ⑨ ⑩ Severe pain

Describe your pain / symptoms

	am	pm
_____	☐	☐
_____	☐	☐
_____	☐	☐
_____	☐	☐
_____	☐	☐
_____	☐	☐
_____	☐	☐

Where does it hurt?

Front   Back

Mood:	🙂 😣 😖 😍 😴 😓 😣 😠
Energy Level:	① ② ③ ④ ⑤ ⑥ ⑦ ⑧ ⑨ ⑩
Stress Level:	① ② ③ ④ ⑤ ⑥ ⑦ ⑧ ⑨ ⑩
Mental Clarity:	① ② ③ ④ ⑤ ⑥ ⑦ ⑧ ⑨ ⑩

Feeling Sick? ☐ Yes ☐ No

☐ Nausea ☐ Vomiting ☐ Congestion ☐ Fever
☐ Diarrhea ☐ Sore Throat ☐ Coughing ☐ Chills

Medications	Time	Dose

Breakfast:

Lunch:

Dinner:

Snacks:

Exercise

☐ None ☐ Stretching ☐ Running/Jogging ☐ Yoga
☐ Walking ☐ Cardio/Weights ☐

Notes:

Made in the USA
Las Vegas, NV
18 December 2024

14633138R00069